"Nutrient Timing represents the next important nutrition concept in the twenty-first century and will teach readers how to optimize their exercise and recovery metabolism to better achieve their fitness and body-development goals."

—William J. Kraemer, Ph.D.
Professor, University of Connecticut

"Drs. Ivy and Portman have made a major contribution to the field of sports nutrition. They've shown that consuming the right nutrients at the right time optimizes the adaptive response of skeletal muscle."

—Jose Antonio, Ph.D., C.S.C.S., F.A.C.S.M.
President, International Society of Sports Nutrition

"The science underlying Nutrient Timing is so strong that a clock will become as important to muscle development as the right training and optimum nutrition."

— Jeff Stout, Ph.D.
Performance Nutrition Consultant

"Nutrient Timing takes the guesswork out of maximizing performance through diet. This book is a must for every athlete."

—Tim N. Ziegenfuss, Ph.D., C.S.C.S.
Chief Scientific Officer, Pinnacle Institute of Health and Human Performance

"This book is a must-read for every strength training athlete and bodybuilder."

—John Berardi, C.S.C.S.
President, Human Performance and Nutrition Counseling

Nutrient Timing System

The revolutionary new system that adds the missing
dimension to optimum sports nutrition—
the dimension of time.

John Ivy, Ph.D., & Robert Portman, Ph.D.

Adapted from Nutrient Timing: The Future of Sports Nutrition

Basic Health PUBLICATIONS, INC.

The information contained in this book is based upon the research and personal and professional experiences of the authors. It is not intended as a substitute for consulting with your physician or other healthcare provider. Any attempt to diagnose and treat an illness should be done under the direction of a healthcare professional.

The publisher does not advocate the use of any particular healthcare protocol but believes the information in this book should be available to the public. The publisher and authors are not responsible for any adverse effects or consequences resulting from the use of the suggestions, preparations, or procedures discussed in this book. Should the reader have any questions concerning the appropriateness of any procedures or preparation mentioned, the authors and the publisher strongly suggest consulting a professional healthcare advisor.

Basic Health Publications, Inc.
8200 Boulevard East
North Bergen, NJ 07047
1-201-868-8336

Library of Congress Cataloging-in-Publication Data
Ivy, John
    Nutrient timing system : the revolutionary new system that adds the missing dimension to sports nutrition : the dimension of time / John Ivy & Robert Portman.—1st ed.
        p. cm.
    Includes bibliographical references and index.
    ISBN 1-59120-146-2
  1. Athletes—Nutrition. I. Portman, Robert II. Title.

    TX361.A8I95   2004
    613.2'024'796—dc22

                                        2004011457

Editor: Carol Rosenberg
Typesetter/Graphics: Gary A. Rosenberg

Printed in the United States of America

10   9   8   7   6   5   4   3   2   1

Contents

Introduction

Nutrient Timing is a revolutionary new system of exercise nutrition that will allow you to build more strength and lean muscle mass in less time than ever before. Its methods are safe and natural, and can be used by anyone—from children to the elderly and from beginning exercisers to professional bodybuilders and power lifters. Nutrient Timing is not a commercial gimmick. Rather, it is the fruit of cutting-edge scientific insights into exercise metabolism, physiology, and nutrition.

The seeds of the Nutrient Timing revolution were planted twenty years ago. Before then, sports nutrition for muscle building and strength training was in the dark ages. It was based on unproven claims, myths, and practices that were not only useless but sometimes even dangerous. There was a feeling that nutrition could help increase muscle strength and lean body mass and stimulate muscle growth, but there wasn't much science to support it.

Hoping to correct this situation, exercise physiologists and nutritionists initiated research studies that measured the effect of increased protein consumption on muscle growth and strength. The results were dramatic. This was the beginning of a revolution in sports nutrition for strength athletes. Old ideas were quickly discarded and a new nutritional paradigm was established. The new paradigm challenged the recommended daily allowance (RDA) for essential nutrients. Protein intake was emphasized and carbohydrate intake de-emphasized. Athletes got results. Thus, "protein" has been the mantra among those involved in resistance training for the last fifteen years.

However, as strength athletes became more intelligent about nutrition and began adopting the new nutrition paradigm with good results, they began to notice what is called the "plateau phenomenon." This phenomenon is characterized by stagnation in muscle strength and growth. Even following the established recommended exercise and diet guidelines did not seem to prevent the plateau phenomenon from occurring.

Eager to tackle this problem, we, along with other colleagues, have become involved in groundbreaking sports-nutrition research. This research adds a new dimension to sports nutrition—the dimension of time. Until now, the strength athlete has focused entirely on *what* to eat. The latest research is providing powerful proof that *when* nutrients are consumed may be even more important. This emerging research on nutrition and how to activate natural anabolic (muscle-building) agents is again changing the way we look at building muscle. These findings form the underpinnings of the next revolution in sports nutrition—Nutrient Timing—which promises to help athletes break through plateaus and achieve higher levels of strength and power.

The easiest way to understand the principles of Nutrient Timing is to look at how the automobile fuel system evolved. In older cars, the primary fuel-delivery device was the carburetor. Older carburetors delivered a crude mixture of oxygen and gasoline to the pistons, which converted this mixture into the power that drives the car. If too much oxygen or gasoline was added to the carburetor, the engine stalled. Carburetors were the standard for almost 100 years, but eventually they gave way to fuel injectors. Fuel injectors are far more efficient in converting oxygen and gas into maximum energy because the mixture is delivered at precisely the time when the piston needs it. Newer cars even have a computer that drives the fuel injectors, making the timing of the delivery of fuel even more precise. As a result, today's cars get better performance out of the same tank of gas.

That's what Nutrient Timing is all about. Until now, strength athletes have used an old carburetor approach to generate muscle growth and energy. The only improvement has been in the type of fuel. We know that certain types of protein are "higher octane" and give better results. But the high-octane protein is still being delivered with imprecise timing by an old "carburetor." By following the principles of Nutrient Timing, you'll be able to deliver the precise amounts of protein and other necessary nutrients at precisely the right time to maximize muscle growth.

Some of the leading sports scientists from the fields of nutrition, exercise physiology, and molecular biology have contributed to these findings. Nutrient Timing is a program built on science. This book includes references to many of the scientific studies related to Nutrient Timing and also provides a list of selected references so that you can review the studies yourself, if you wish.

The exciting new science of Nutrient Timing will enable you to achieve more dramatic results in muscle growth and strength than you ever thought possible. Nutrient Timing will enable you to minimize muscle damage and soreness after a hard workout, and your "plateau phenomenon" will become just a bad memory. By applying the principles of Nutrient Timing, you can actually sculpt a better body with more lean muscle mass, less fat, and more power without changing your exercise program or even your total caloric intake.

Nutrient Timing is, above all, a practical program. The information in this book will change the way you look at nutrition and, more important, change the results you get from your hard time in the gym. We'll show you specifically how to apply the latest findings to change the way your body builds muscle, burns fat, and stores energy for the next workout.

As scientists, we are excited about these findings. As athletes, we are applying them to our own programs and have experienced results firsthand. Nutrient Timing is the future of sports nutrition. Read on to learn how to make it work for you.

Nutrient Timing

During a muscle's twenty-four-hour growth cycle, there are periods when the muscle is actively involved in producing energy, periods when it is recovering, and periods when it is growing. For the metabolic machinery of the muscle to function at its best during each of these periods, the appropriate amounts and types of nutrients must be consumed at the appropriate times.

Depending on its metabolic needs at any given time, the muscle machinery can be directed to produce and replenish muscle glycogen (the stored form of glucose) or synthesize muscle protein. Each of these operations requires different types of nutrients, and if you're able to deliver the right nutrient mixture to the muscles at the right time, you can greatly enhance recovery from exercise and improve muscle growth, strength, and power.

To understand why Nutrient Timing is such a revolutionary concept, we must first take a look at sports nutrition over the past twenty years. The focus of sports nutrition has been on the types of nutrients that are best for the strength athlete. It was quickly recognized that strength athletes need more protein than is recommended for the average person and that an increased consumption of protein could improve muscle development.

This has led to a "bulk nutrition" mentality. If protein is good, then more protein must be better. Unfortunately, you can consume the protein of an entire cow, but if your muscles are not receptive at that particular time, the protein will be wasted. And, in fact, the evidence indicates that very few strength athletes fail to get enough protein to support muscle growth. Then why do so many athletes plateau in their training? The answer lies in *when* nutrients are consumed, which is what Nutrient Timing is all about. By consuming the same amount of nutrients, but keying your consumption to the three phases of muscle growth discussed below, you will be able to avoid the plateau effect and achieve far greater gains in muscle strength and muscle mass.

THE THREE PHASES OF THE NUTRIENT TIMING SYSTEM (NTS)

There are three phases of the Nutrient Timing System: the Energy Phase, the Anabolic Phase, and the Growth Phase.

The Energy Phase

The Energy Phase coincides with your workout. The primary metabolic objective of the muscle during this phase is to release sufficient energy to drive muscle contraction. Most athletes recognize the importance of consuming carbohydrates during exercise both to prevent depletion of muscle glycogen stores, which helps extend endurance, and to maintain blood glucose levels, which helps delay fatigue. Nutrient Timing, however, entails more than just consuming carbohydrates during exercise. Research has shown that when you consume carbohydrates with protein, specific amino acids, and vitamins, you will be able to spare muscle glycogen and achieve greater muscular endurance, blunt the rise in the catabolic hormone cortisol (thereby reducing muscle damage), and help prepare your muscle enzymes for a faster recovery following your workout.

The Anabolic Phase

The Anabolic Phase is the forty-five-minute window following a workout in which your muscle machinery, in the presence of the right combination of nutrients, initiates the repair of damaged muscle protein and replenishes muscle glycogen stores. Immediately after exercise, muscle cells are extremely sensitive to the anabolic effects of the hormone insulin. This sensitivity, however, declines rapidly, and, after several hours, muscle cells even become insulin resistant. Insulin resistance is a condition that dramatically slows muscle glycogen recovery, repair of existing muscle, and synthesis of new muscle.

As you read this book, you will come to understand why consumption of carbohydrates during this time period is so important for driving muscle glycogen recovery and muscle tissue repair and synthesis. You'll also learn why protein consumed without carbohydrate is far less efficient during the Anabolic Phase. Moreover, you'll learn why specific antioxidants such as vitamins C and E and amino acids can speed muscle recovery.

The Growth Phase

The Growth Phase extends from the end of the Anabolic Phase to the beginning of the next workout. It is the time when the muscle enzymes are involved in increasing the number of contractile proteins and the size of muscle fibers, as well as in helping the muscle fully replenish muscle glycogen depleted during the Energy Phase. During the Growth Phase, consumption of carbohydrate and protein is essential to maintain optimal muscle growth. The latest research shows that a high intake of protein can be of significant benefit to the strength athlete if protein is consumed at the correct time. By following the Nutrient Timing System, you'll be able to maintain a high anabolic state and restore muscle glycogen, repair muscle tissue damage, and synthesize new muscle.

IMPORTANT CONCEPTS IN THE NUTRIENT TIMING SYSTEM

The Nutrient Timing System is going to challenge much of what you've been taught to believe about exercise nutrition. For the past twenty years, nutritionists, exercise physiologists, and strength athletes have painted nutrients in black-and-white terms: "Sugar is bad and protein is good." These generalized prejudices may be useful in building an overall healthy diet, but they often don't take into account the metabolic realities of muscle cells during and after exercise.

Following are three true statements that most strength athletes would find pretty hard to believe. They illustrate important concepts in the Nutrient Timing System.

"A low-quality protein can be more effective in stimulating protein synthesis than a high-quality protein."

Everything that you have heard or read would suggest that the above statement is false. The shelves of health food stores are filled with products proclaiming their superiority because they contain a better-quality protein. However, the effectiveness of any protein product is largely dependent on *when* you take it.

Muscles can modify their metabolic activity in response to changing needs and various stimuli at any given instant. This is called "metabolic sensitivity." A good example is the effect of the hormone insulin. If insulin is stimulated when you are not exercising, it can cause a conversion of carbohydrate into fat, which is the last thing a strength athlete needs. However, in the forty-five minutes after a workout (the Anabolic Phase), the metabolic machinery of the muscle is extremely sensitive to insulin. Insulin has been shown to drive the rebuilding, or anabolic activity, of the muscle. Nutrients consumed during this postexercise "metabolic window" are much more effective than those consumed later, when the muscle becomes insulin resistant.

Let's look at our shocking but true statement in the light of Nutrient Timing. Consuming a poor-quality protein, such as corn, during the forty-five-minute postexercise metabolic window will actually result in greater protein synthesis than consuming a high-quality protein, such as whey protein isolate, two hours later. And the difference is not small. The high-quality protein consumed two hours later may result in 85 percent less protein synthesis compared with the corn protein taken immediately after the workout.

"Sugar can stimulate protein synthesis."

For strength athletes, "sugar," or carbohydrate, is the poster boy for bad nutrition. Nutrition articles in bodybuilding and strength-training publications routinely discuss the negative effects of carbohydrates. Much of what they say is true—up to a point. Unfortunately, your muscle cells do not read articles appearing in the popular press. This brings us to the second essential concept of Nutrient Timing. It's called "nutrient activation."

Your muscle cells never rely on a single nutrient. Rather, muscle metabolism is a tightly scripted symphony involving fat, carbohydrate, protein, vitamins, minerals, and water. The proportions of nutrients consumed can significantly affect the degree to which you are able to achieve the results you are seeking. Consuming too much carbohydrate may result in increased body fat. Consuming too much protein or consuming it at the wrong time may produce no benefit except to the manufacturers of protein powders.

An excellent example of nutrient activation is the addition of simple (high-glycemic) sugars to protein. Studies have shown that a high-glycemic carbohydrate/protein supplement can dramatically enhance protein synthesis. In fact, in one study, a high-glycemic carbohydrate/protein drink was 38 percent more effective in stimulating protein synthesis than a conventional protein drink.

The reason for this effect is that the high-glycemic carbohydrates can serve as nutrient activators. Consuming high-glycemic carbohydrates following exercise stimulates insulin, one of the most important regulators of protein synthesis following exercise. When insulin is stimulated in the presence of protein, the result is greater synthesis of new protein. In other words, carbohydrates prime the protein pump by first stimulating insulin. A complex carbohydrate is less effective because it is a weaker stimulator of insulin.

By now you may be thinking that this book is about the benefits of carbohydrates. It is not. But there are certain times—namely during and immediately following workouts—when the addition of simple carbohydrates can have dramatic effects on the muscle cells' anabolic processes, which can lead to greater increases in muscle strength and endurance.

"Sugar is more effective than protein in preventing protein degradation in the muscle."

The third important concept in the Nutrient Timing System is "nutrient optimization." The consumption of certain nutrients at specific times not only can help the muscle recover faster, but can also shift the metabolic machinery from a catabolic state into an anabolic one. Following strenuous exercise, there is a significant increase in blood cortisol levels. Cortisol is the enemy of strength athletes because it breaks down muscle protein; however, its release is a normal part of the body's response to the stress of exercise. By consuming carbohydrates during exercise, you can reduce the cortisol response and thereby lessen protein breakdown. Consumption of high-glycemic sugars increases blood insulin levels. Among its many effects, insulin prevents protein degradation. Thus, by increasing insulin levels postexercise in the presence of other essential nutrients such as protein, you can turn off the muscle's catabolic switch and turn on its anabolic one.

You may still be skeptical. However, we encourage you to reserve final judgment until you've read more about the Nutrient Timing System. We will challenge some of your long-held beliefs and introduce you to many new ideas about exercise and nutrition. You'll find that the bulk theory of protein consumption gives you a false sense of accomplishment and may even hinder muscle development. You'll learn about the critical metabolic window during which you have an opportunity to double or triple protein synthesis. You'll learn how carbohydrates can increase blood flow to your muscles, and you'll find out why two small helpings of protein may be more effective than a single large helping. Nutrient Timing can also show you how to reduce your susceptibility to colds and infection.

Finally, you will soon realize that the Nutrient Timing System is a simple one. You won't have to walk around with a stopwatch timing every meal to the last millisecond. All you'll have to do is recognize that there are critical times during and after exercise to stimulate the muscle's natural anabolic agents. Best of all, you'll see the results almost immediately.

Table 1.1 on the following page explains when the three Nutrient Timing phases fall in relation to your daily workout and the benefits of consuming the right combination of nutrients within each phase. Chapter 2 describes the metabolic processes that take place in the three phases of your muscles' growth cycle and why nutrient intervention can play a critical role. And in Chapter 6, we show you how to easily incorporate the Nutrient Timing System into your own training program.

TABLE 1.1. Nutrient Timing System (NTS) Phases and Goals

NTS Phase	Time	What NTS Can Do for You
ENERGY	10 minutes prior to and during a workout	Increase nutrient delivery to muscles and spare muscle glycogen and protein
		Limit immune system suppression
		Minimize muscle damage
		Set the nutritional stage for a faster recovery following your workout
ANABOLIC	Within 45 minutes after a workout	Shift metabolic machinery from a catabolic state to an anabolic state
		Speed the elimination of metabolic wastes by increasing muscle blood flow
		Replenish muscle glycogen stores
		Initiate tissue repair and set the stage for muscle growth
		Reduce muscle damage and bolster the immune system
GROWTH	**Rapid Segment** The first 4 hours after a workout	Maintain increased insulin sensitivity
		Maintain the anabolic state
	Sustained Segment The next 16–18 hours after a workout	Maintain positive nitrogen balance and stimulate protein synthesis
		Promote protein turnover and muscle development

Hormones— The Regulators of Nutrient Timing

Every athlete who does resistance exercise knows at least a little bit about hormones. They are the agents that drive muscle development. In general, athletes classify hormones as good (anabolic) or bad (catabolic). But this is too simplistic. Even the so-called "bad" hormones are essential because they break down nutrients that provide the energy to drive muscle contraction. Even the "good" ones often stimulate reactions, such as increased fat deposition, that are not considered beneficial to the strength athlete.

Hormones are chemical messengers. In response to certain stimuli, they are released from one organ and travel via the bloodstream to another (the target organ), where they initiate a specific cell reaction. Both catabolic and anabolic hormones are important for resistance training. Anabolic hormones stimulate rebuilding and repair reactions in the muscle. Catabolic hormones stimulate the breakdown of carbohydrate, fat, and even protein for energy.

Using the principles of Nutrient Timing, you will learn how to turn on the anabolic hormones, and, at the same time, turn off the catabolic ones to maximize muscle growth and development.

Cortisol—The Primary Catabolic Hormone

Cortisol is well known by strength athletes. This hormone is released from the adrenal glands when blood glucose is low and during very intense exercise such as weightlifting. Cortisol's major function is to generate fuel for working muscles. During exercise, your muscles use a metabolic priority system for generation of energy. This is particularly true during aerobic exercise. First, carbohydrate is used, then fat, and finally protein. Because of the tremendous stress that resistance training places on the muscles, the metabolic priority system gets ignored. When cortisol is released, it causes a breakdown of protein, carbohydrate, and fat and an increase in plasma amino acids, specifically glutamine and the branched-chain amino acids (BCAAs).

Elevated cortisol levels have enormous implications for strength athletes. The harder the workout is, the greater the cortisol release, and the greater the resulting protein degradation. Cortisol is the reason that many strength athletes reach a plateau. The anabolic benefits of exercise can actually be negated by the catabolic effect of cortisol.

Insulin—The Primary Anabolic Hormone

Insulin may be the most misunderstood hormone among strength athletes because of its association with carbohydrate. High levels of insulin combined with high carbohydrate intake have been shown to increase fat synthesis and decrease fat breakdown. Chronic elevation of blood insulin levels maintained over many years with the resulting accumulation of body fat is associated with type II (adult-onset) diabetes.

However, while it's true that high levels of insulin promote fat synthesis, they do not necessarily do so to the same degree in all circumstances. Insulin is just as effective in promoting carbohydrate fuel storage and muscle protein synthesis. The degree to which insulin promotes fat storage, carbohydrate storage, or protein synthesis at any given time depends on certain aspects of the individual's body state. Perhaps the most important factor is the relative degree of insulin sensitivity in fat cells versus muscle cells: the more insulin sensitive the fat cells are at a given time, the more insulin will act to promote fat storage; the more insulin sensitive the muscle cells are, the more insulin will act to promote muscle glycogen storage and protein synthesis.

Muscle cells are especially insulin sensitive after exercise. If glucose and amino acids are made available at this time, insulin will help synthesize muscle proteins and muscle glycogen at a very rapid rate, and very little fat will be synthesized and stored in adipose (fat) tissue.

Lifestyle factors can increase the insulin sensitivity of the muscle cells and thereby create a body that is generally disposed to build muscle proteins and less disposed to store body fat. Exercise and a moderate-carbohydrate diet that is rich in fiber can increase muscle insulin sensitivity. Alternatively, a low-carbohydrate, high-fat diet can decrease insulin sensitivity, which, as you will soon see, can have negative effects on muscle mass and strength.

Because of its many actions, insulin has earned the title "anabolic regulator of the muscle." In fact, insulin may be the most important hormone to increase muscle strength and mass. Insulin is also at the heart of the Nutrient Timing System.

Insulin is released from the pancreas usually in response to high levels of blood glucose. Most people are familiar with the fact that insulin increases the transport of glucose into the muscle cell, but insulin plays many more roles, as you will quickly learn.

INSULIN INCREASES PROTEIN SYNTHESIS

Insulin has a number of actions that increase protein synthesis. Insulin stimulates DNA and RNA, thereby increasing the enzymes responsible for protein synthesis. Researchers from the University of Texas Health Science Center in Galveston found that, following an insulin infusion, protein synthesis in the muscle cell increased almost 67 percent.

INSULIN INCREASES AMINO ACID TRANSPORT

Although most people are aware that insulin increases glucose transport into muscle cells, most are not aware that insulin also increases amino acid uptake into the muscle. This is important because amino acids are the building blocks of protein. Muscle cell enzymes need a sufficient supply of amino acids to drive protein synthesis. Insulin has been shown to increase the rate of transport of key amino acids into the muscle from 20 percent to 50 percent and this increase was associated with enhanced protein synthesis.

INSULIN REDUCES PROTEIN DEGRADATION

Net protein gain is a function of protein synthesis and protein degradation. Net protein gain will occur whenever protein synthesis exceeds protein degradation. Even though there is a strong increase in protein synthesis after exercise, there is also considerable protein degradation. In fact, there is actually a net protein loss. By decreasing protein degradation, we can change this net protein reduction into a net protein gain. Insulin suppresses protein degradation following exercise, thereby increasing net protein gain.

INSULIN INCREASES GLUCOSE UPTAKE

Insulin's ability to increase glucose uptake is its best-known action. Following exercise, the metabolic machinery is involved in replenishing muscle glycogen. Insulin shuttles glucose into the muscle where it can then be converted into glycogen by muscle cell enzymes. After exercise, the muscle is very receptive to insulin stimulation of glucose uptake.

INSULIN INCREASES MUSCLE GLYCOGEN STORAGE

During resistance exercise, muscle glycogen stores can be significantly reduced. Aside from creatine phosphate (CP), glycogen is the primary fuel for the replenishment of ATP. The conversion of glucose into glycogen takes place via the activation of the enzyme glycogen synthase. Following exercise, insulin can increase the activity of glycogen synthase by 70 percent, resulting in a tremendous increase in glycogen storage.

INSULIN SUPPRESSES CORTISOL RELEASE

The primary trigger for cortisol release during prolonged aerobic exercise is hypoglycemia, or reduced blood glucose levels. This is to be expected, since hypoglycemia is a metabolic stress to the nervous system. Therefore, it is also not surprising that carbohydrate supplementation during exercise would blunt the rise in cortisol, and this cortisol-blunting action appears to be mediated by insulin. Higher insulin concentrations protect muscle protein from the catabolic effects of cortisol.

Insulin's effect on cortisol may also help maintain immune function. Colds and other viral infections are quite common in athletes undergoing intensive training. Cortisol has been shown to suppress the immune system and antibody production. Thus, the cortisol-blunting effects of insulin may also help keep athletes healthy.

INSULIN INCREASES MUSCLE BLOOD FLOW

Another, less well-known but essential effect of insulin is on muscle blood flow. Insulin infusion has been shown to increase skeletal muscle and limb blood flow by more than 100 percent. Insulin not only increases muscle blood flow, but it targets specific muscles that have been exercised. Increased blood flow results in faster removal of metabolic wastes, such as lactic acid and carbon dioxide, and an increased delivery of nutrients, such as amino acids, glucose, and oxygen, for a more rapid recovery from exercise.

SUMMARY

Hormones are the regulators that drive nutrient timing. Contrary to popular belief, insulin is the most powerful anabolic hormone—the most important hormone of all in relation to muscle growth. It is not all good all the time, however. If you are sedentary and have a high-carbohydrate diet, insulin can increase fat stores. But if you are a strength athlete who trains smart and practices the Nutrient Timing System correctly, you will find yourself harnessing the great power of insulin to achieve your goal of gaining muscle mass and strength and keeping your body fat level very low.

NTS Energy Phase

The Energy Phase of the Nutrient Timing System is the period of your workout. The objective of a resistance workout is to repeatedly require the muscles to generate high levels of force, which requires a high rate of energy release. This chapter explains how the principles of Nutrient Timing will help you produce the energy needed to achieve a stronger workout, how to minimize muscle damage that occurs as a natural consequence of exercise, and, most important, how to set the stage for a faster recovery following your workout.

PHYSIOLOGICAL AND METABOLIC CHANGES DURING EXERCISE

Exercise stresses many systems of the body. At the onset, there is an immediate need to produce greater amounts of energy; as exercise intensity increases, so do the muscles' energy requirements. To accommodate these increased energy needs, the body must initiate multiple physiological and metabolic changes. While these changes are essential for providing an adequate supply of energy to the working muscles, they may also result in transient adverse effects such as muscle damage and immune system suppression. Let's consider some of the more important changes and their consequences.

ATP Replenishment

Muscle fibers need a rapid supply of energy during a resistance workout. This requires the utilization of large numbers of ATP molecules. The breakdown of ATP releases the energy that directly drives muscle contraction. There is, however, only enough ATP stored in the muscle for a few seconds of maximal effort. Therefore, ATP has to be rapidly and continuously replenished during repetitive or sustained muscle contractions.

The primary sources for rapid repletion of ATP during intense exercise are creatine phosphate (CP) and muscle glycogen. Unfortunately, CP stores in the muscle are also quite limited and are depleted with just ten to twelve seconds of maximum-intensity work. If you combine the amount of ATP stored in the muscle and the amount of CP available to replenish ATP, you have only enough energy to drive exercise for twelve to eighteen seconds.

The rapid repletion of ATP and CP involves the anaerobic energy system, or glycolysis. In the anaerobic energy system, muscle glycogen is broken down to generate ATP. Most strength athletes do not realize how much muscle glycogen is used during a training session. One set of ten biceps curls results in a 12 percent loss of muscle glycogen; three sets result in 35 percent depletion, and six sets result in 40 percent depletion.

Hormonal Changes

During resistance exercise there are changes in a number of key hormones. Anabolic hormones such as testosterone, growth hormone, and IGF-1 are elevated for a short period of time and are not believed to play a major role during exercise. There is also a rise in epinephrine and norepinephrine, two catabolic hormones that increase the breakdown of muscle glycogen and fat for energy.

The two most important regulatory hormones during exercise are insulin and cortisol. The opposing actions of these two hormones affect the degree of muscle damage and glycogen depletion during exercise. In the absence of nutritional supplementation, insulin levels decline during exercise while levels of cortisol begin to rise.

Blood Flow

Because of the increased energy and nutrient needs of the muscle, blood flow to active muscles is elevated up to 500 percent. This elevated blood flow results in faster delivery of oxygen and fuel and faster removal of metabolic wastes such as lactic acid and carbon dioxide.

Effect on the Protein Pool

During sustained exercise, a net muscle protein loss occurs. This is mainly because there is an increased use of branched-chain amino acids (BCAAs) for energy. BCAAs are generated by muscle protein breakdown. Because BCAAs serve as precursors for the synthesis of glutamine, muscle glutamine stores decline as well. Glutamine, the most abundant amino acid in muscles, plays an important role in providing fuel for the immune system. During prolonged stressful exercise, glutamine stores can be almost completely depleted, potentially compromising immune system function.

Muscle Damage

Muscle damage is perhaps the most significant physiological effect of a resistance workout. Exercise physiologists measure muscle damage by using a number of key biochemical markers such as 3-methylhistidine, creatine phosphokinase (CPK), and lactate dehydrogenase (LDH). Because 3-methylhistidine is only found in the muscle contractile protein, its presence in the urine indicates that the muscle fibers have been damaged. Like 3-methylhistidine, CPK and LDH are usually found only within the muscle fiber but appear in the blood when muscle fiber membranes are damaged.

There is no single cause of exercise-related muscle damage. The three primary causes are physical, hormonal, and biochemical. Initial damage occurs as a result of physical forces acting on the muscle cell. Eccentric exercise, in which muscle fibers lengthen while contracting, places great stress on the muscle fibers, resulting in an overstretching and tearing of the contractile proteins, which can lead to inflammation. Some of this damage may be beneficial since it stimulates remodeling of muscle cell fibers, which ultimately results in strength and mass gains. William Kraemer of the University of Connecticut coined the term *muscle tissue disruption* to describe this type of damage because the muscle tissue can recover within twenty-four hours and isn't compromised in its ability to adapt to training.

The second cause of muscle damage is hormonal—specifically, the hormone cortisol stimulates muscle protein breakdown.

The third cause of muscle damage is the generation of free radicals (highly reactive molecules that can damage muscle protein). Free radicals may come from the mitochondria, from the capillaries, or even from specific types of cells associated with the immune system. Regardless of their origin, free radicals can damage cell membranes and may indirectly inactivate key enzymes associated with proper functioning of the immune system.

Acute Inflammatory Response

The acute inflammatory response is the body's response to tissue injury, whether it's caused by exercise, an ankle injury resulting from a fall, or even a cut. Within hours of an injury, specific cells called neutrophils migrate to the site of the damage, where they begin to remove tissue debris. This process causes inflammation and swelling, which further damage muscle cell membranes. The acute inflammatory response continues for a considerable period of time after exercise (which is one reason why muscle soreness often isn't felt for twenty-four hours or more).

Immune Response

Resistance exercise triggers a strong immune response. The immune system responds anytime there is cellular damage, whether it is caused by a virus, a wound, or exercise. The immune system's response to the different types of injuries is quite similar. There is an increase in white blood cells, an increase in natural killer (NK) cells, and an increase in T cells, important fighters of infection. However, during strenuous exercise, there is suppression of the immune system as evidenced by a decrease in the number of T cells and NK cells. This suppression has been found to be intensity- and duration-related. The higher the relative exercise intensity and the longer it is performed, the greater the suppression of the immune system. Immune system suppression can last up to seventy-two hours following exercise and may increase your susceptibility to infection.

Fluid Loss

Water, of course, is a vital nutrient that serves many functions. It is the major constituent of blood. Consuming water during exercise helps maintain blood volume, lower body temperature, and reduce stress on the heart. For the endurance athlete, because dehydration represents the number one physiological risk during exercise, the number one nutritional objective is fluid replacement. For an endurance athlete, a loss of 2 percent body water (3.6 pounds for a 180-pound athlete) will compromise performance. In sports such as football, basketball, and soccer, fluid losses exceeding 2 percent of body weight are frequently observed.

Resistance exercise does not produce fluid losses to the degree that extended aerobic exercise does, but dehydration is still a factor. In a study from Old Dominion University, researchers found that dehydration equal to a 1.5 percent loss of body weight adversely affected strength performance.

Most athletes now recognize the benefits of hydration and even carbohydrate replenishment while training. However, it should now be quite obvious that the metabolic processes occurring during resistance exercise require more intensive nutrient intervention. Even water with carbohydrates (for example, a typical sports drink) just doesn't meet the complete nutrient needs of working muscles.

NTS GOALS FOR THE ENERGY PHASE

The four primary goals of the Nutrient Timing System during the Energy Phase are:

1. Increase nutrient delivery to muscles and spare muscle glycogen and protein.

2. Limit immune system suppression.

3. Minimize muscle damage.

4. Set the nutritional stage for a faster recovery following your workout.

1. Increase Nutrient Delivery to Muscles and Spare Muscle Glycogen and Protein

Although glycogen depletion has traditionally been the concern of endurance athletes, it is also an important issue for strength athletes. Muscle glycogen levels following multiple sets can be reduced as much as 40 percent. Doubling the intensity of the workout doubles the breakdown.

ATP and creatine phosphate provide most of the energy for muscle contraction, but glycolysis still plays an important role. Between sets, muscle cells use the glycolytic pathway to regenerate ATP. By consuming a carbohydrate or carbohydrate/protein sports drink during your workout, you can preserve muscle glycogen and remain strong throughout your workout.

Researchers have found that when carbohydrate supplementation is provided during resistance exercise, the decline in muscle glycogen was 50 percent less and that subjects could perform more work than subjects receiving flavored water.

The latest research now shows that the addition of protein to a carbohydrate supplement during resistance exercise offers further advantages in terms of preserving muscle protein, increasing protein synthesis, and even extending endurance.

During extended exercise, amino acids—principally the BCAAs: leucine, isoleucine, and valine—may supply up to 15 percent of the muscles' energy needs. The use of some BCAAs for energy can be increased by as much as 500 percent, depending on the intensity and duration of the exercise. The addition of protein to a carbohydrate supplement promotes the metabolism of the ingested protein and lessens the demand for amino acid release from the muscles.

Recent studies coming out of the University of Texas Health Science Center in Galveston suggest that when protein is added to a carbohydrate supplement and provided at the beginning of exercise, there is even an increase in protein synthesis after exercise.

Finally, the addition of protein to a carbohydrate supplement has been shown to extend muscular endurance. Researchers from the University of Texas in Austin found that a carbohydrate/protein drink improved endurance 57 percent compared with water and 24 percent compared with a carbohydrate-electrolyte drink (see Figure 3.1). The improvement in endurance was thought to be due to a sparing of muscle glycogen and possibly to the preferential metabolism of the ingested protein.

2. Limit Immune System Suppression

A second objective of the NTS during the Energy Phase is limiting immune system suppression. During moderate-intensity exercise, immune function is heightened, increasing resistance to infection. However, as discussed, with strenuous exercise, the immune system is suppressed, and the risk of infection is thereby increased.

The immune system is closely linked to the neuroendocrine system, which controls the release of hormones. During strenuous and sustained exercise, this system is activated, causing the release of cortisol. Most of the immunosuppressive responses caused by intense exercise correlate with increases in blood cortisol levels. Cortisol lowers the concentration and activities of many of the important immune cells that fight infection.

Interestingly, blood cortisol levels can be regulated to a signif-

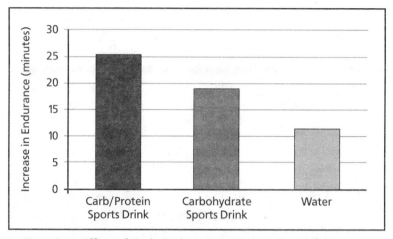

Figure 3.1. Effect of Carbohydrate/Protein Supplementation During Exercise
Following variable intensity exercise, subjects receiving a carbohydrate/protein sports drink had a 24 percent improvement in exercise endurance compared with a carbohydrate sports drink and a 57 percent improvement compared with water. *(Adapted from Ivy et al.)*

icant degree during exercise by controlling glucose availability. When athletes were given a 6 percent carbohydrate solution during exercise, cortisol levels dropped by almost 80 percent compared with subjects receiving water (see Figure 3.2).

Because of the high correlation between cortisol and immune system suppression, it is logical that carbohydrate supplementation would limit the suppressive effects of exercise on the immune system. This has been confirmed by researchers at Appalachian State University who compared a number of immune system parameters during exercise with and without carbohydrate supplementation. They found that subjects receiving carbohydrate supplementation during intense exercise had lower blood cortisol levels and limited immune suppression—as indicated by a lessened T cell and NK cell reduction—compared with subjects receiving a placebo.

Carbohydrate supplementation provides a dual benefit during

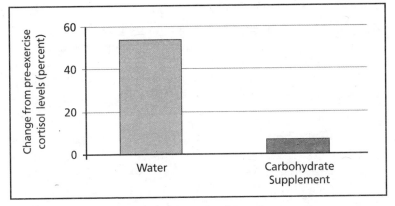

Figure 3.2. Effect on Cortisol Levels of Supplementation During Exercise
When athletes were administered a 6 percent carbohydrate solution during exercise, blood cortisol levels dropped almost 80 percent. *(Adapted from Bishop et al.)*

exercise. It helps maintain immune function while decreasing cortisol levels.

During resistance exercise, cortisol levels can increase fivefold. Strength athletes who ignore the benefits of nutrient supplementation during their workouts place themselves at a greater risk of experiencing the immune-suppressive effects of cortisol, which include a transient weakening of the body's major mechanisms of fighting infection.

3. Minimize Muscle Damage

The third important objective of Nutrient Timing during the Energy Phase is to reduce muscle damage. This damage is beneficial to a degree because it stimulates the remodeling process, which leads to larger and stronger muscles. However, the damage to the muscles must be repaired before the remodeling process can begin. Because there is no single cause of exercise-related muscle damage, nutritional intervention must address all the causes.

Carbohydrate supplementation during exercise has been

shown to reduce the rise in cortisol and decrease specific agents responsible for producing inflammation by almost 50 percent.

Supplementation with the antioxidant vitamins E and C and BCAAs may also help minimize muscle damage. While there does not appear to be a performance benefit from vitamins C and E, supplementation with these antioxidants decreases levels of CPK, an important marker of muscle damage, twenty-four hours after a marathon. This finding suggests that they may limit tissue damage due to free radicals. Dr. William Evans from the University of Arkansas, a leader in this area, has suggested that antioxidants may be of benefit in the body's overall response and adaptation to exercise.

4. Set the Nutritional Stage for a Faster Recovery Following Your Workout

An important tenet of the Nutrient Timing System is nutritional intervention at all stages in the muscle's growth cycle. Increased muscle mass comes from a cycle of muscle stimulation, muscle breakdown, and muscle rebuilding. Every athlete knows the expression *No pain, no gain*. This is true in the sense that you must train hard enough to cause a degree of muscle tissue disruption. However, training hard without appropriate nutrition intervention results in a more prolonged recovery and ultimately a weaker training response.

Although you cannot entirely prevent muscle damage and depletion of your energy stores during resistance exercise, by applying the principles of the Nutrient Timing System you can minimize these effects, setting the stage for a faster recovery.

As seen above, there is increased muscle protein degradation, in part to help supply muscle energy needs during exercise. Consuming protein during exercise will enable you to utilize the ingested protein and thereby decrease protein degradation and spare muscle protein. The same principle holds true with regard to muscle glycogen. Consuming carbohydrate during resistance exercise results in less depletion of glycogen stores.

The replenishment of muscle glycogen stores is an essential cellular function that is given a metabolic priority by the muscles' anabolic machinery following exercise. The faster this replenishment process occurs, the quicker the muscle machinery can be reoriented toward the remodeling of your muscle fibers. The replenishment of your energy stores occurs much faster if you have limited their depletion during your workout by supplementing appropriately.

NTS RECOMMENDATIONS FOR THE ENERGY PHASE

Now that you recognize the importance of nutrient consumption during the Energy Phase, we would like you to redefine when your workout actually begins. For most, it begins with your warm-up stretching or first weightlifting repetition. But there are a number of benefits to be gained if you begin your workout instead while you are driving to the gym. Consumption of a carbohydrate/protein drink ten minutes prior to your workout can raise both blood glucose and insulin levels. At the beginning of your workout, there will be an increase in glucose uptake into the muscles for use as energy, resulting in greater sparing of muscle glycogen and an increase in endurance. A second benefit is that consumption of a carbohydrate/protein drink immediately *before* exercise results in greater protein synthesis *after* exercise. A third potential benefit is that by raising the blood glucose level, you may reduce the rise in cortisol, which begins soon after your workout does.

Nutrient supplementation immediately before exercise and continuing every fifteen to twenty minutes during exercise will not only improve your workout but also lay the groundwork for a faster recovery. Water will help replenish fluid, but a carbohydrate drink or, even better, a carbohydrate/protein drink will deliver additional benefits. If you are to take full advantage of the Nutrient Timing System, the ideal drink to consume before and during exercise should contain the ingredients specified in, and described following, Table 3.1.

TABLE 3.1. Ideal Nutrient Composition of Supplement for the Energy Phase		
NTS OBJECTIVE	**Nutrient**	**Amount** (per 12 oz water)
• Increase nutrient delivery to muscles and spare muscle glycogen and protein	High-glycemic carbohydrates such as glucose, sucrose, and maltodextrin	20–26 g
	Whey protein	5–6 g
• Limit immune system suppression	Leucine	1 g
	Vitamin C	30–120 mg
• Minimize muscle damage	Vitamin E	20–60 IU
	Sodium	100–250 mg
• Set the nutritional stage for a faster recovery following your workout	Potassium	60–100 mg
	Magnesium	60–120 mg

Carbohydrate

Carbohydrate supplementation during exercise not only helps extend endurance, but also limits suppression of the immune system and reduces muscle tissue damage. The ideal carbohydrates to use are high-glycemic ones such as sucrose, glucose, and maltodextrin. Drinks that contain large quantities of fructose may cause gastrointestinal problems.

Protein

Consuming protein during your workout will limit muscle protein degradation. Protein can also work synergistically with carbohydrate to increase blood insulin levels beyond those produced by carbohydrate alone. Protein has been shown to extend exercise endurance and to increase protein synthesis upon cessation of exercise. The protein of choice is whey because it is rapidly absorbed and contains all the essential amino acids, as well as a high percentage of leucine and glutamine, two amino acids that are used extensively during sustained strenuous exercise. The ratio of carbohydrate to protein should be approximately 3–4 grams of carbohydrate to 1 gram of protein, as this formulation is highly digestible.

Leucine

This amino acid may also be of benefit in a sports drink because it not only stimulates insulin in its own right, but also has a positive effect on protein synthesis.

Electrolytes

Sodium, potassium, and chloride are also necessary in an effective sports drink. The addition of electrolytes not only helps replace what's lost due to sweating but also encourages continued fluid consumption because of the salt, which stimulates thirst.

Vitamins

Although many sports drinks contain varying amounts of different vitamins, we recommend adding vitamins E and C because they reduce free-radical levels, an important cause of muscle damage.

Fluids

You should try to fully replace fluid and electrolyte losses that occur during a strength-training workout. Although strength training does not produce the same level of fluid loss as an endurance workout, fluid losses can still be considerable. Drink at least 12 ounces starting ten minutes before and continuing throughout your workout. For maximum effectiveness, consume several ounces of your Energy Phase beverage every fifteen minutes. In warm weather or when conditions are hot, increase your beverage consumption accordingly.

NTS Anabolic Phase

The Anabolic Phase is the most critical phase of the Nutrient Timing System. Following a workout, the muscle machinery is primarily in a catabolic mode. However, it is primed to switch into an anabolic mode if the right stimuli are provided.

The principles of nutrient optimization and metabolic sensitivity are particularly relevant during the forty-five-minute period post-exercise. The switch that turns off the catabolic machinery and turns on the anabolic machinery is insulin. During this forty-five-minute period, muscle cells are acutely sensitive to the anabolic actions of insulin. Just providing the right nutrients will exploit this insulin sensitivity and cause a tremendous surge of anabolic activity.

First, let's consider what happens once we stop exercising. Following exercise, the state of the muscle in many ways is similar to that seen during exercise; however, if recovery measures are not taken, this state can actually worsen. ATP and creatine phosphate (CP) levels are depleted, muscle glycogen levels are reduced, and the rise in cortisol seen during exercise continues in the post-exercise period, which means that there is heightened catabolic activity. Other catabolic hormones, such as epinephrine and nor-epinephrine, remain elevated for thirty to sixty minutes and then return to pre-exercise levels. On the other hand, free radicals generated during exercise are present and will attack muscle cell structure, causing damage for many hours after exercise.

The muscle damage that occurred during exercise has stimulated an acute inflammatory response. Specific cells migrate to the site of muscle damage, increasing inflammation and releasing specific proteins that cause additional damage to muscle membranes. Markers of muscle damage like CPK actually reach a peak twenty-four hours after a workout—further evidence that membrane damage continues in the postworkout period.

As the damaged muscle cell attempts to repair and rebuild, the increase in protein synthesis that you would expect has been observed. However, the rate of protein degradation exceeds the rate of protein synthesis, resulting in a net muscle protein loss. Furthermore, unless specific nutritional actions are taken, this catabolic state can continue for a considerable period of time.

Some essential amino acids, glutamine, and branched-chain amino acids (BCAAs) are also depleted. This depletion is believed to occur because of the use of amino acids in vital metabolic processes. Because BCAAs are a precursor for glutamine synthesis, their use as an energy source may result in lower glutamine levels.

If the above reasons don't arouse your concern about the state of your muscles postexercise, there is one more. Elevated blood flow postexercise supports the rapid removal of metabolic byproducts and faster nutrient and oxygen delivery. Unfortunately, this is a transitory elevation; blood flow quickly returns to its normal resting level, even though the recovering muscle still requires greater oxygen and nutrient delivery.

Considering this fuel depletion and the biochemically compromised state of the muscles following a workout, it is somewhat surprising to look at what a strength athlete typically consumes during recovery. For many, it is just water. For others, it may be a protein drink. Although each provides a benefit, neither is adequate for complete recovery.

THE METABOLIC COST OF NUTRIENT DELAY

The forty-five minutes immediately following exercise (the Anabolic Phase) is the metabolic window of opportunity. At no other time during the course of your day can nutrition make such a major difference in your overall training program. Although the muscle has residual catabolic activity following exercise, it is primed to shift into an anabolic state in the presence of the right nutrients. If you don't exploit this metabolic receptivity, your muscle cells will remain in a catabolic state and even begin to develop insulin resistance. The metabolic window is only open for a short period of time after exercise. Indeed, within minutes after you stop exercising, it begins to close.

Taking in more nutrients outside the metabolic window will not produce the same results. When insulin resistance develops, usually two to four hours after your workout, even the perfect combination of nutrients will be much less effective.

TIMING AND GLYCOGEN REPLENISHMENT

As early as 1988, researchers from the University of Texas at Austin showed that the timing of carbohydrate supplementation post-exercise had a significant influence on the rate of muscle glycogen storage. They found that when subjects consumed a carbohydrate supplement immediately after exercise, they stored twice as much muscle glycogen in a two-hour recovery period as when they took the same supplement two hours later. Similar results were obtained by researchers at Vanderbilt University, who found that muscle glucose uptake following exercise was three to four times faster when supplementation was given immediately after exercise rather than three hours later.

TIMING AND PROTEIN SYNTHESIS

Stimulation of protein synthesis is essential for all strength athletes. The ineffectiveness of the bulk protein philosophy (more is better) is illustrated when the relationship between timing and optimal protein synthesis is closely examined.

In order for protein synthesis to occur, amino acids must be transported into the cell, where they can be utilized by the metabolic machinery to repair, rebuild, and remodel muscle protein. Muscle amino acid uptake is controlled in part by the blood amino acid levels. In addition, the level of amino acids in the blood is a critical initiator of protein synthesis. Research studies show that when the amino acid levels of the blood are reduced to below normal, amino acids are released from the muscle and muscle protein synthesis declines. When the blood amino acid levels are increased above normal, muscle amino acid uptake increases as does muscle protein synthesis.

Activation of protein synthesis by amino acids is most responsive immediately following exercise. Amino acid uptake and muscle protein synthesis is threefold greater in subjects who have engaged in resistance exercise compared with subjects who have not. Researchers have also found that in the postexercise recovery period, protein synthesis was almost 25 percent higher and amino acid uptake almost twice as high when a carbohydrate/protein supplement was given immediately after exercise versus two hours after exercise.

The importance of consuming protein during the Anabolic Phase, however, is best illustrated by the results of a study at Vanderbilt University. These researchers looked at the effect of a carbohydrate/protein supplement on protein synthesis following a sixty-minute bout of exercise. Subjects were given the supplement immediately after exercise or three hours later. Protein synthesis was almost three times higher when the supplement was given immediately after, compared with a three-hour waiting period. And the all-important net protein balance (protein synthesis minus protein degradation) increased significantly in the immediate group. In the three-hour group there was actually a net loss of protein. (See Figure 4.1.)

Besides the benefit of increased protein gain, the group receiving the carbohydrate/protein supplement immediately after exercise also had greater fat oxidation—that is, they burned more fat.

TIMING AND INCREASED MUSCLE MASS

Although supplement timing is critical for protein synthesis and net protein balance, it is also important for muscle development.

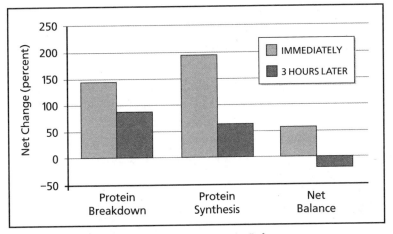

Figure 4.1. Effect of Delay on Net Protein Balance
Subjects were given a carbohydrate/protein supplement either immediately following exercise or three hours after exercise. Receiving supplementation immediately after exercise resulted in an increase in net protein balance, whereas receiving the supplementation three hours after exercise resulted in a net protein loss. *(Adapted from Levenhagen et al.)*

After all, a major goal of most strength athletes is to increase muscle mass.

Using laboratory animals, scientists investigated the effects of Nutrient Timing on body composition. They found that when animals were fed right after exercise versus four hours later, muscle weight was higher by 6 percent in the group fed immediately. They also reported that the muscle enzymes responsible for fat oxidation were 70 percent higher and abdominal fat was 24 percent lower in the group immediately fed. The researchers suggested that, compared with nutrient supplementation several hours later, the consumption of nutrients after exercise may contribute to an increase in muscle mass and a decrease in adipose (fat) tissue.

Similar results were seen in a recent human trial. In a twelve-week training study, researchers reported that when a carbohydrate/protein mixture was given immediately after each exercise session, muscle size increased 8 percent and strength improved 15 percent. When the supplement was given two hours later, there was no muscle hypertrophy (growth) or improvement in strength.

The evidence is overwhelming. Consumption of nutrients during the Anabolic Phase can help you replenish glycogen stores faster, increase protein synthesis and net protein balance, improve muscle mass, and even speed up fat oxidation. But not just any nutrients will do. Although drinking a sports drink is preferable to drinking water, consuming that alone will cost you a great opportunity to improve muscle development. You must consume all of the critical nutrients in the right proportions while the metabolic window is open.

The two conditions for muscle growth are metabolic sensitivity and nutrient optimization. The first condition is satisfied in the postexercise interval because your muscle cells are ready to begin the rebuilding and recovery process. For nutrient optimization, all you have to do now is consume all of the nutrients necessary to drive recovery.

NTS GOALS FOR THE ANABOLIC PHASE

The five goals of the Nutrient Timing System during the Anabolic Phase are:

1. Shift metabolic machinery from a catabolic state to an anabolic state.

2. Speed the elimination of metabolic wastes by increasing muscle blood flow.

3. Replenish muscle glycogen stores.

4. Initiate tissue repair and set the stage for muscle growth.

5. Reduce muscle damage and bolster the immune system.

All of this sounds pretty complicated, but it's not. Once again, the science shows that these goals are readily achievable by following some simple steps.

1. Shift Metabolic Machinery from a Catabolic State to an Anabolic State

In Chapter 3, you learned how important insulin is in regulating anabolic processes. Now, the most effective way to stimulate insulin release is to ingest high-glycemic sugars, right? Not exactly. While ingesting carbohydrate alone will accomplish the goal, it is nowhere near as effective as using a carbohydrate/protein supplement.

Use of a carbohydrate/protein supplement will stimulate insulin and blunt cortisol release. The synergistic effects of carbohydrate and protein were first noted almost forty years ago. In an effort to determine the effect of food on insulin secretion, scientists noted that foods high in protein, when combined with carbohydrates, raised blood insulin levels more than other food combinations or carbohydrate alone.

Researchers at the University of Texas at Austin extended these findings by comparing the effects of carbohydrate, protein, and carbohydrate/protein supplements on blood insulin levels after exhaustive exercise. The carbohydrate/protein drink produced the greatest insulin response followed by the carbohydrate drink and then the protein drink. (See Figure 4.2.) In fact, the protein supplement by itself produced one-eighth as much insulin response as the carbohydrate/protein combination. Not only did the carbohydrate/protein produce a greater response, but it was also found that this response could be maintained throughout the recovery period with continued supplementation to drive post-workout anabolic processes.

Stimulating insulin release is the first step in shifting the metabolic machinery to an anabolic state after exercise. Once high levels of insulin are achieved, a number of anabolic reactions are activated in the presence of the right nutrients.

2. Speed the Elimination of Metabolic Wastes by Increasing Muscle Blood Flow

Recovering muscle requires fast nutrient and oxygen delivery as

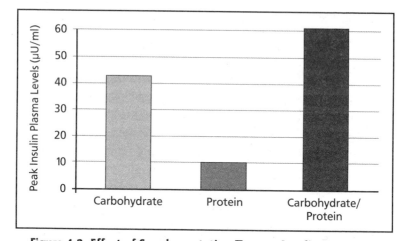

Figure 4.2. Effect of Supplementation Type on Insulin Response
Effect of carbohydrate, protein, and carbohydrate/protein supplementation on blood insulin levels after exhaustive exercise. A carbohydrate/protein supplement produced the greatest insulin response. *(Adapted from Zawadzki et al.)*

well as fast removal of metabolic byproducts such as lactic acid. Removal of lactic acid is particularly important to the recovery of creatine phosphate (CP), the main precursor by which ATP is regenerated during resistance exercise. When lactic acid levels are high, it takes longer for CP to be restored. Insulin has been shown to increase skeletal muscle blood flow approximately twofold (see Figure 4.3).

The mechanism by which insulin increases skeletal muscle blood flow involves nitric oxide synthesis. Nitric oxide (NO) has lately received a lot of attention as a means to induce vasodilation (increased blood flow) in muscle. The precursor for NO is the amino acid arginine. A number of arginine products are currently available from manufacturers who tout their ability to increase NO production. Studies suggest that insulin is also a strong stimulator of the NO pathway. In one study, insulin infusion into the blood was shown to be more effective in increasing NO-dependent muscle blood flow than 30 grams of arginine.

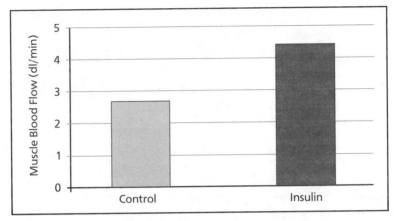

Figure 4.3. Effect of Insulin on Muscle Blood Flow
Following insulin infusion, muscle blood flow almost doubled when compared with muscle blood flow in a control group. *(Adapted from Laasko et al.)*

3. Replenish Muscle Glycogen Stores

Some of the most important studies on exercise recovery have measured the effects of carbohydrates on the replenishment of muscle glycogen stores postexercise. These studies have found that supplementing with carbohydrate immediately after exercise is much more effective than delaying supplementation. It has also been found that supplementing on a regular basis after exercise can maintain a rapid rate of glycogen storage during the early hours of recovery, and that carbohydrates that produced the greatest insulin response also produce the highest rates of glycogen storage. In fact, the rate of muscle glycogen storage postexercise appears to be directly related to the blood insulin response. That is, the higher the insulin response the greater the rate of muscle glycogen synthesis.

Trying to increase the blood insulin level by simply increasing the carbohydrate content of the supplement was initially effective, but only up to a point. When the carbohydrate content of the supplement exceeded 0.5 grams of carbohydrate per pound of body weight per hour, both the blood insulin response and the rate of muscle glycogen synthesis plateaued.

After this plateau effect was discovered, a number of investigators, knowing that by stimulating a greater amount of insulin they would probably also stimulate a stronger surge in anabolic activity, began to investigate whether they could increase the level of insulin by adding one or more additional nutrients to carbohydrates.

In a pivotal study performed at the University of Texas at Austin, researchers demonstrated that adding protein to a carbohydrate supplement could increase the effectiveness of the carbohydrate to stimulate muscle glycogen synthesis by increasing the blood insulin response. The carbohydrate/protein supplement was found to be almost 38 percent more effective in restoring muscle glycogen than a carbohydrate supplement and almost four times more effective than a protein supplement. Using nuclear magnetic resonance spectroscopy, a sophisticated technique that evaluates the rate of muscle glycogen storage, these researchers also showed that a carbohydrate/protein supplement was significantly more effective than a carbohydrate supplement of equal caloric content. Interestingly, during the first forty-five minutes of recovery, muscle glycogen storage for the carbohydrate/protein supplement was two times faster than the carbohydrate supplement containing the same amount of calories.

In another study comparing the effects of a carbohydrate/protein drink to those of a carbohydrate drink, scientists at Maastricht University in the Netherlands found a near doubling of the insulin response to the former that was consistent with a near doubling of muscle glycogen storage.

The importance of rapidly replenishing muscle glycogen was clearly evidenced in a collaborative study that included researchers from North Texas State University School of Medicine and the University of Texas at Austin. When subjects consumed a carbohydrate/protein drink, endurance performance after four hours of recovery was 55 percent greater than when they consumed a carbohydrate drink (see Figure 4.4). The increase in performance

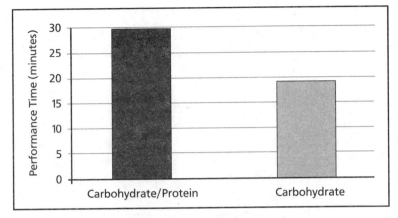

Figure 4.4. Effect of Postworkout Supplementation on a Subsequent Exercise Bout
Following a glycogen-depleting exercise bout, subjects were given either a carbohydrate or a carbohydrate/protein/antioxidant/glutamine beverage. Following a four-hour recovery period, the subjects completed an exercise bout to exhaustion. When the subjects received the carbohydrate/protein/antioxidant/glutamine drink, their performance times in the second workout were 55 percent better than when they received the carbohydrate supplement. *(Adapted from Williams et al.)*

was directly related to greater muscle glycogen synthesis during the recovery period. Researchers in the Allied Health Science Center at Springfield College have also documented faster recovery and better performance in a subsequent workout when comparing carbohydrate/protein and carbohydrate supplements.

4. Initiate Tissue Repair and Set the Stage for Muscle Growth

Because net protein gain is a sum of both synthesis and breakdown, merely looking at protein synthesis as a measure of net protein gain can be misleading. To increase muscle mass and strength in the postworkout period, the muscle cell must begin to initiate tissue repair and to set the stage for muscle growth.

Researchers at McMaster University in Hamilton, Ontario,

reported that supplementing with a carbohydrate supplement, both immediately and one hour after resistance exercise, increased muscle protein synthesis. They noted higher blood insulin and glucose levels and lower 3-methylhistidine excretion following consumption of the carbohydrate supplement. You may recall that 3-methylhistidine excretion is an indicator of muscle fiber damage.

However, a carbohydrate/protein supplement had a greater effect on postexercise protein synthesis. Investigators from Vanderbilt University showed that a carbohydrate/protein supplement provided immediately after exercise increased protein synthesis almost sixfold over a carbohydrate supplement. The results for the all-important net protein balance were even more telling. The carbohydrate/protein supplement showed a significant increase in net protein balance compared with the carbohydrate supplement.

Intuitively, you might expect these results since protein synthesis requires amino acids, which obviously are not found in a carbohydrate supplement. A more interesting comparison would be between a carbohydrate/protein supplement and a protein supplement. The answer to this question comes from a recent study from the University of Texas Health Science Center at Galveston. Scientists evaluated the effects of a carbohydrate supplement, an amino acid supplement, and an amino acid/carbohydrate supplement on protein synthesis. The results were dramatic. As shown in Figure 4.5, the researchers found that protein synthesis was greatest with the carbohydrate/amino acid supplement and least with the carbohydrate supplement. In fact, the carbohydrate/amino acid supplement was 38 percent more effective than the amino acid supplement and 100 percent more effective than the carbohydrate supplement. This study, more than any other study, should convince you that that the combination of carbohydrate and protein produces a synergistic effect on protein synthesis.

Consumption of a carbohydrate/protein drink postexercise may also replenish glutamine stores faster. In one study, plasma

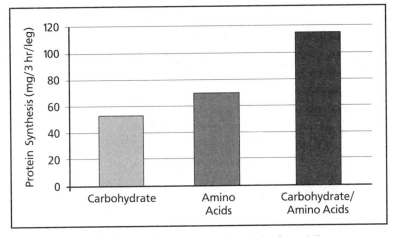

Figure 4.5. Effect of Amino Acids and Carbohydrate Mixture on Protein Synthesis Following Exercise
Following resistance exercise, subjects received either a carbohydrate, amino acid, or carbohydrate/amino acid supplement. The carbohydrate/amino acid mixture increased protein synthesis 38 percent more than the amino acid mixture and 100 percent more than the carbohydrate supplement. *(Adapted from Miller et al.)*

glutamine levels decreased 20 percent in subjects receiving the carbohydrate alone and remained low in recovery. In subjects consuming the carbohydrate/protein supplement, postexercise glutamine levels did not decline.

5. Reduce Muscle Damage and Bolster the Immune System

The final goal of Nutrient Timing in the Anabolic Phase is to reduce muscle damage and stimulate the immune system. There is no way to eliminate all the muscle damage resulting from resistance exercise. In fact, to do so would even be undesirable since muscle damage serves as a stimulus for muscle growth. However, excessive muscle damage will restrict glycogen and protein synthesis, cause excessive muscle soreness, and delay recovery. Therefore, to the degree that you can limit muscle damage and reduce muscle soreness, you can come back stronger the next day. Here again, nutrition in the postexercise period plays a role. Using a carbohydrate/protein drink that also contained vitamins E and C and glutamine, researchers found a significant reduction in free-radical formation compared with a plain carbohydrate supplement.

Using this same multi-nutrient beverage composition, researchers at St. Cloud University reported a 37 percent reduction in blood CPK, an important marker of muscle damage, after a prolonged exercise bout (see Figure 4.6).

One of the most exciting examples of how nutrition can reduce muscle inflammatory responses and positively impact the immune system comes from a recent collaborative study conducted by researchers from Iowa State, Vanderbilt University, and the United States Marine Corp. The researchers looked at the effect of placebo (no nutrients), a carbohydrate control, and a carbohydrate/protein supplement taken by Marine recruits after exercise over a

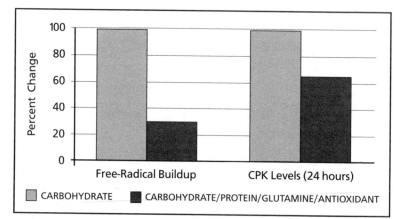

Figure 4.6. Effect of a Carbohydrate/Protein Drink Containing Antioxidants and Glutamine on Parameters of Muscle Damage
Subjects were given either a carbohydrate or a carbohydrate/protein/glutamine/antioxidant supplement immediately after exercise. Free radicals were reduced 69 percent and CPK levels were reduced 36 percent at twenty-four hours postexercise.

fifty-four-day period. Individuals receiving the carbohydrate/protein supplement experienced:

- 33 percent fewer total medical visits.
- 28 percent fewer visits due to bacterial/viral infections.
- 37 percent fewer visits due to muscle joint problems.
- 83 percent fewer visits due to heat exhaustion.

The researchers suggested that the effect of postexercise supplementation with a carbohydrate/protein supplement on the immune system may be related to the increased availability of specific amino acids such as glutamine, and concluded that the postexercise carbohydrate/protein supplement "may not only enhance muscle protein deposition but also has significant potential to positively impact health, muscle soreness and tissue hydration."

NTS RECOMMENDATIONS FOR THE ANABOLIC PHASE

One important takeaway from this chapter is this: Don't wait if you intend to take full advantage of the postexercise recovery window. This is clearly evidenced in Figure 4.7, which summarizes the effects of delayed nutrient supplementation on muscle anabolic activities. Almost every important anabolic activity is reduced after three hours.

Another important lesson is that any nutrition taken during this interval is better than just plain water. However, the Nutrient Timing System is about optimizing muscle growth and development. The studies described in this chapter show that you will receive many more benefits if your postexercise meal contains the right combination of nutrients. Here are the nutrients/supplements we recommend during the Anabolic Phase.

Whey Protein

Whey protein offers a number of advantages. It contains all nine essential amino acids. It is extremely digestible. It has a higher concentration of BCAAs than any other protein source. It is fast acting

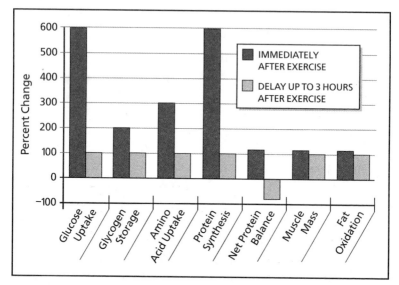

Figure 4.7. Effect of Nutrient Delay on Muscle Anabolic Processes
A delay in nutrient supplementation of up to three hours can dramatically decrease important anabolic activities including glycogen storage
and protein balance.

because it empties from the stomach and is absorbed into the
bloodstream faster than other proteins. It also contains precursors
for the body's natural antioxidants, which may help minimize
free-radical formation. Whey protein is readily available and relatively inexpensive.

A disadvantage of whey protein is that it contains lactose.
However, lactose-free whey-protein products, which contain lactose amounts of less than 1 percent, are now available.

High-Glycemic Carbohydrates

High-glycemic carbohydrates, which are rapidly absorbed and
produce a strong insulin response, are far preferable to complex
carbohydrates, which are absorbed far more slowly. Remember,
high-glycemic carbohydrates are the catalysts that drive higher
anabolic activity postexercise. High-glycemic carbohydrates ideal

for postexercise supplementation include sucrose, maltodextrin, and dextrose. Avoid products containing a high percentage of fructose or galactose. These products are weaker stimulators of insulin.

Carbohydrate/Protein Ratio

Studies show conclusively that a carbohydrate/protein combination is superior in stimulating both glycogen replenishment and protein synthesis to either a carbohydrate or protein supplement alone. Carbohydrate provides a strong stimulus for insulin but also provides substrate for replenishment of muscle glycogen stores. The many studies involving carbohydrate/protein supplements that have been cited in this chapter used different ratios of carbohydrate and protein. Based on a review of these studies, we recommend a 3:1 to 4:1 ratio of high-glycemic carbohydrates to protein—in other words, 3 to 4 grams of carbohydrate per gram of protein. Table 4.1 compares the effects of different beverages on key metabolic activities following a workout. This table, which synthesizes the findings of many different studies, makes a very compelling case for a carbohydrate/protein supplement as the only way to go.

Amino Acids

Amino acids not only serve as a driving force for protein synthesis postexercise, but specific ones such as leucine and glutamine have additional properties that can help in the muscle-recovery process. Leucine, by itself, helps stimulate protein synthesis. Glutamine is also an excellent candidate for inclusion in a postworkout drink because muscle glutamine stores are depleted following heavy exercise and glutamine has been shown to play an important role in maintaining a healthy immune system.

Antioxidants

Antioxidant vitamins such as E and C should also be included. A hard workout produces free radicals, which not only cause muscle protein damage but also may even have a negative effect on the body's immune system.

ADDITIONAL CONSIDERATIONS FOR THE ANABOLIC PHASE

Although nutrient supplementation can be taken in the form of a meal or beverage, we know full well that after a hard workout most athletes simply are not hungry. However, if they wait until they are hungry, they will miss the critical forty-five-minute window. In our experience, a beverage is easier to consume; therefore, we have formulated the ideal beverage. The beverage should contain between 220 and 260 calories. For most athletes, this amount of energy can be consumed in 12 ounces of water. This guideline works well for athletes weighing up to 170 pounds. Athletes who weigh more should increase the amount by 50 percent. Table 4.2 provides the ingredient composition for the ideal supplement to consume during the Anabolic Phase.

TABLE 4.1. Relative Comparison of Different Beverages Used Postexercise (Anabolic Phase)

Functional Activity	Water	Carbohydrate/ Electrolyte	Protein	Carbohydrate/ Protein/ Electrolyte/ Antioxidant
Restore fluids	√	√	√	√
Restore electrolytes		√		√
Replenish glycogen		√		√√
Stimulate protein synthesis		√	√√	√√√
Increase amino acid uptake			√	√√
Prevent protein degradation		√		√√
Blunt cortisol		√		√
Maintain glutamine levels			√	√√
Stimulate insulin		√√	√	√√√
Bolster immune function		√	√	√√
Reduce muscle damage		√	√	√√

TABLE 4.2. Ideal Nutrient Composition of Supplement for the Anabolic Phase		
NTS OBJECTIVE	**Nutrient**	**Amount**
• Shift metabolic machinery from a catabolic state to an anabolic state	Whey protein	13–15 g
	High-glycemic carbo-hydrates such as glucose, sucrose, and maltodextrin	40–50 g
• Speed the elimination of metabolic wastes by increasing muscle blood flow	Leucine	1–2 g
• Replenish muscle glycogen stores	Glutamine	1–2 g
• Initiate tissue repair and set the stage for muscle growth	Vitamin C	60–120 mg
• Reduce muscle damage and bolster the immune system	Vitamin E	80–400 IU

NTS Growth Phase

The third phase of the Nutrient Timing System is the Growth Phase. This is the eighteen- to twenty-hour period during which the majority of gains in muscle mass and strength occur. Life would be easier for strength athletes if the muscles' anabolic machinery operated in a consistent manner for the full interval between workouts. Unfortunately, this is not the case. There are two discrete time segments within the Growth Phase that can be characterized by the intensity of anabolic activity.

The first, the Rapid Segment, is a period of high anabolic activity, which lasts up to four hours if activated during the Anabolic Phase. The second is the Sustained Segment in which muscle growth continues but at a slower rate. This phase is mainly influenced by your diet.

First let's review what happens to muscles following the Anabolic Phase, the forty-five minutes that follow your workout.

When supplementation does not occur, blood insulin levels will remain low and blood cortisol levels will be elevated. Muscle glycogen will remain depleted. Protein degradation and muscle membrane damage will continue. There is continued damage from free radicals and suppresion of the immune system. But the most important change is that without nutrient intervention muscles start to go from a state of high insulin sensitivity to a state of insulin resistance. Once insulin resistance develops, the ability of your muscle cells to maximize anabolic activity, even in the presence of the right nutrients, is severely compromised. When the cellular machinery becomes insulin resistant, which starts about two hours after exercise, it can continue for sixteen hours or longer.

Now let's assume you recognize the importance of postexercise nutrition and have consumed a carbohydrate/protein drink containing glutamine, leucine, and antioxidants immediately after your workout. So you have done everything right. You have increased the blood insulin level, reduced the blood cortisol level, and turned on the anabolic switch. Now you can relax while the cellular machinery of your muscles replenishes the muscle glycogen stores, repairs damaged tissue, and increase muscle protein. Right?

Unfortunately, this is not what happens. Again, to use the car-engine analogy, in the Anabolic Phase you have turned on the cellular ignition and placed the transmission in forward, but if you don't provide sufficient fuel, your car will soon run out of gas. In this case, running out of gas means running out of enough carbohydrate and protein (amino acids) to maintain an elevated blood insulin level, and stimulate muscle glycogen and protein synthesis. Only by keeping insulin levels elevated can high rates of glycogen storage and protein synthesis be maintained during the Rapid Segment.

RAPID SEGMENT OF THE GROWTH PHASE

An important aspect of Nutrient Timing is that, although the muscle growth cycle occurs in separate phases, in reality supplementation in each phase influences the subsequent phase. Turning on the anabolic switch during the Anabolic Phase is the essential first step, but without continuing the right type of nutrient consumption, this anabolic surge will not be maintained.

The two NTS objectives for the Rapid Segment of the Growth Phase are:

1. Maintain increased insulin sensitivity.

2. Maintain the anabolic state.

1. Maintain Increased Insulin Sensitivity

Researchers at the University of Texas at Austin showed that the ability of the muscle cell to replenish glycogen stores is 50 percent less two hours after exercise than it is immediately after exercise. Investigators at Vanderbilt University have reported similar results for protein synthesis. When a carbohydrate/protein supplement was given immediately after exercise, muscle protein synthesis was elevated 300 percent, but when the supplement was delayed by three hours, the elevation in synthesis was only 12 percent. These results indicate that the muscle is more insulin sensitive early in the recovery period, and that as time passes, it becomes insulin resistant.

Once the muscle becomes insulin resistant, as we have seen, consuming the right nutrients will not produce the desired effect. In other words, the anabolic processes necessary to rebuild and help the muscles grow will not operate at their optimal rate. This means that additional carbohydrates must be consumed with protein and other essential nutrients. However, this becomes a delicate nutritional balance. You want to consume only enough carbohydrates to make sure that the insulin pump is primed and muscle sensitivity to insulin is not lost.

A review of the literature suggests that in the Anabolic Phase, supplements should be composed of a 3:1 to 4:1 ratio of carbohydrate to protein (3 to 4 grams of carbohydrate per gram of protein) to fully convert the muscle from a catabolic state to an anabolic state. During the Rapid Segment of the Growth Phase, you can capitalize on the insulin response that was initiated during the

Anabolic Phase. The question is, what is the ideal quantity of carbohydrate to be added to protein?

The muscles in the typical strength athlete have between 100 grams and 120 grams of glycogen per kilogram of muscle. During a strenuous high-intensity workout, about 40 percent of this stored glycogen will be depleted. If you consume sufficient carbohydrate and protein during the Anabolic Phase, as much as 65 to 75 percent of your glycogen stores are replenished within two hours of completing your workout, with no additional supplementation.

Once this level of glycogen storage is attained, a lower consumption of carbohydrate in conjunction with protein will provide sufficient stimulus to keep blood insulin levels elevated. This will maintain the muscle cells' sensitivity to the anabolic effects of insulin and assure complete recovery of muscle glycogen.

During the Energy and Anabolic Phases, it is almost mandatory that insulin be strongly stimulated to drive protein synthesis and muscle recovery. Figure 5.1(a) illustrates the twenty-four-hour cycle of insulin sensitivity in the muscle in the absence of any supplementation during or after exercise. As you can see, muscles are extremely sensitive to insulin during exercise. This sensitivity decreases without any nutrient intervention and muscles actually become insulin resistant two hours after exercise. This insulin-resistant state can last up to sixteen hours after exercise if nutrient intake is withheld.

Figure 5.1(b) illustrates the goal of nutrient intervention. Consumption of a carbohydrate/protein sports drink during exercise and a carbohydrate/protein recovery drink postexercise prevents the development of insulin resistance, allowing the muscle cells to maintain a high level of anabolic activity. To the degree that you can extend the muscles' insulin sensitivity for up to three to four hours after the Anabolic Phase, you will be rewarded with greater gains in lean muscle mass and strength. It is important to remember that the goal is not to keep blood insulin levels high for the full twenty-four-hour growth cycle. This would not be beneficial. But if you can maintain elevated blood insulin and muscle insulin sen-

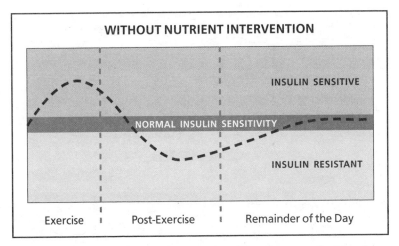

Figure 5.1(a). The Effect of Exercise and Recovery on the Muscle Response to Insulin (without Supplementation)
In the absence of supplementation, the muscles' sensitivity to insulin decreases rapidly. During the postexercise period, muscles become insulin resistant and can remain so for up to sixteen hours if nutrient intake is withheld.

sitivity during the Rapid Segment, the benefits to your muscle-development program will be substantial.

2. Maintain the Anabolic State

The second objective is to maintain the anabolic state for up to four hours after exercise. Researchers found that providing a high-carbohydrate supplement immediately after exercise and continuing supplementation at two hours and again at four hours after exercise maintained a high blood insulin level and rapid rate of muscle glycogen synthesis for up to six hours.

A similar pattern was seen with regard to protein synthesis where scientists studied the effects of consuming a carbohydrate/protein drink at one hour and again at three hours after a bout of resistance exercise. When the carbohydrate/protein drink was consumed at one hour, there was a sharp rise in insulin, which

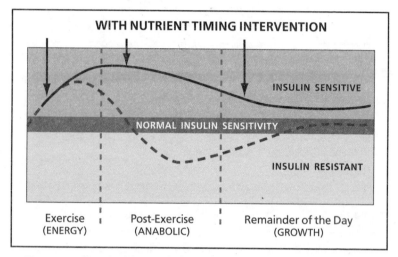

Figure 5.1(b). The Effect of Nutrient Timing on the Muscle Response to Insulin

When nutrient supplementation is supplied during the Energy Phase, Anabolic Phase, and Rapid Segment of the Growth Phase, muscle cells are insulin sensitive for an extended period of time. This extended insulin sensitivity in the presence of nutrient intervention enables the muscle cells to maintain a high level of anabolic activity.

returned to resting values within one hour. The researchers also found that protein synthesis only increased during the time when insulin was elevated. Thus, the stimulation and decline of protein synthesis paralleled blood levels of insulin. When a second serving of the carbohydrate supplement was given at three hours postexercise, blood insulin rose once again and protein synthesis was stimulated back to its peak levels.

One of the first studies to investigate the long-term effects of maintaining an active anabolic state after exercise comes from Japanese researchers. In their study, they fed a high-glycemic carbohydrate and protein meal to animals undergoing ten weeks of resistance training. One group of animals received their first meal of the day during the first hour after their exercise session, and the second group of animals received their first meal of the day during the

fourth hour after their exercise session. After the ten weeks of training, there was no difference in weight gain between the two groups
of animals; however, muscle mass was 6 percent higher and body
fat 25 percent lower in the group fed immediately after exercise.
Interestingly, the animals fed immediately after exercise had a higher resting metabolic rate, possibly due to their greater muscle mass.

Leucine may also be helpful in maintaining high anabolic
activity during this time. A study conducted at the University of
Illinois found that leucine stimulates muscle protein synthesis following exercise. The effect of leucine on protein synthesis appears
to be independent of its effects on insulin. However, when insulin
was stimulated by carbohydrate in combination with leucine,
there was a further increase in protein synthesis. The authors suggested that leucine in combination with carbohydrate would be
useful in helping muscles recover faster.

SUSTAINED SEGMENT OF THE GROWTH PHASE

This segment begins approximately five hours after exercise
and continues until your next workout. The time you are
sleeping is included in this segment. Your total diet is criti-
cally important during this phase. The two NTS objectives
for the Sustained Segment of the Growth Phase are:

1. Maintain positive nitrogen balance and stimulate protein
synthesis.

2. Promote protein turnover and muscle development.

1. Maintain Positive Nitrogen Balance and Stimulate Protein Synthesis

An essential condition of muscle growth is the maintenance of a
positive nitrogen balance. This means that your body is excreting
less protein than you are consuming. How much protein does one

need to consume in order to maintain a positive protein balance? This is a controversial question. Some nutritionists maintain that the average diet contains more than enough protein for the serious strength athlete. According to the recommended daily allowance (RDA), protein intake should be 0.8 grams per kilogram (2.2 pounds) of body weight per day. The problem is that the nutritionists who developed this recommendation were using sedentary adults as their models. Furthermore, they were not suggesting that this level of protein intake maintains a positive nitrogen balance (positive protein retention), but rather that it maintains a zero nitrogen balance. That is, the amount of protein consumed would prevent a net protein loss, but would not necessarily allow for protein gain.

How much protein should be consumed daily? Obviously, the goal of the strength athlete is not to be in zero nitrogen balance, but to be in positive nitrogen balance. In this regard, investigators have shown that a high protein intake will increase nitrogen balance in strength athletes during intense training. Interestingly, a review of the available data indicates that 20 percent of the protein consumed in excess of the maintenance amount is retained. In other words, when a greater amount of protein is ingested, lean body mass is increased. A positive nitrogen balance can be maintained for up to fifty days on a diet that is three times the RDA for protein.

So how much protein do we recommend? Researchers found a greater gain in muscle mass over four weeks of training in bodybuilders who consumed 3.3 grams versus 1.3 grams of protein per kilogram of body weight per day. This suggests that large amounts of dietary protein in combination with strength training will stimulate significant muscle growth. It was also noted that when the bodybuilders consumed the higher protein concentration, a significant amount was oxidized and not retained. This suggests that protein intake exceeded that which could be used for protein synthesis.

An increase in whole-body protein synthesis was observed

when strength athletes increased their protein consumption from 0.9 to 1.4 grams per kilogram (g/kg) of body weight per day. However, there was no additional increase in protein synthesis when protein consumption was increased to 2.4 g/kg of body weight per day. Additionally, other researchers have reported that approximately 1.5 g/kg of body weight per day were required to maintain zero nitrogen balance in strength athletes undergoing intense training. Having a positive nitrogen balance required approximately 1.8 g/kg of body weight.

Recently, scientists compared the twenty-four-hour macronutrient metabolism of subjects who had exercised and were on either a high-protein diet (2.5 g/kg of body weight per day) or a normal protein diet (1 g/kg of body weight per day). They found the subjects on the high-protein diet had a positive protein balance and negative fat balance, whereas the subjects on the normal protein diet had zero protein balance and a slight increase in fat balance. In other words, the subjects on the high-protein diet burned more fat.

Based on these studies, we concluded that the strength athlete will receive significant benefits from consuming between 2.0 and 2.75 grams of protein per kilogram of body weight (0.9–1.25 gram of protein per pound of body weight) per day when training intensely. This should be a sufficient amount of protein to maintain a positive nitrogen balance, stimulate muscle growth, and increase reliance on body fat as a fuel source. To make it easy for you to determine your daily protein intake use, Table 5.1 provides the daily protein requirements at protein levels ranging from 0.91–1.25 grams per pound of body weight per day for different body weights.

2. Promote Protein Turnover and Muscle Development

During the Sustained Segment of the Growth Phase, it is important to continue to promote protein turnover and muscle development. Protein turnover is an essential process in helping build stronger

Weight	Daily Protein Level (grams per pound)			
(in pounds)	0.91	1.02	1.14	1.25
125	114	128	143	156
150	137	153	171	188
175	159	179	200	219
200	182	204	228	250
225	205	230	257	281
250	228	255	285	313

TABLE 5.1. Grams of Protein Required According to Body Weight in Pounds

muscles. By definition, protein turnover involves both the processes that break down protein and the processes that build new protein. The reason that protein turnover is an important NTS objective is that when protein turnover is increased, you are rebuilding proteins damaged by training. The result is stronger muscles containing more muscle fibers.

Although protein synthesis will be slower during this segment than during the Rapid Segment, there is still a substantial amount of protein accretion (an increase in protein concentration within a muscle) that can occur during the Sustained Segment of the Growth Phase. Protein synthesis may continue after exercise for up to forty-eight hours. However, as we have seen, net protein balance remains negative unless the appropriate foods or amino acid supplements are consumed.

During the Sustained Segment, it is important to maintain elevated blood levels of amino acids, as shown in Figure 5.2. This can be done by eating a meal high in protein and snacking between meals with a protein supplement. Researchers have found a positive relationship between the concentration of amino acids in the blood and the rate of protein synthesis. Their results show that increasing protein consumption will increase amino acid levels in the blood and lead to increased protein synthesis.

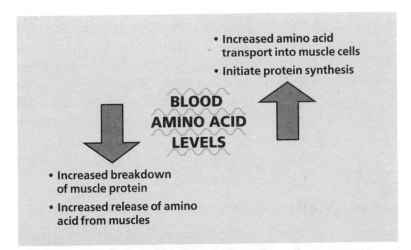

Figure 5.2. Effect of Blood Amino Acid Level on Protein Synthesis and Breakdown

An increase in blood amino acids stimulates amino acid transport into the muscle and increases protein synthesis. When blood amino acid levels are low, there is an increased breakdown of muscle protein and a decrease in overall protein synthesis.

Snacking between meals may be advantageous for several reasons. Results from the University of Texas Health Science Center in Galveston showed that increasing blood amino acid levels improved protein synthesis, but only up to a certain point. After that, the protein-synthesis response failed to increase proportionately. Thus, consuming your protein in one large meal may be much less effective in stimulating muscle protein synthesis than consuming a normal meal and snacking between meals with a high-protein supplement.

In order to maintain a rapid protein turnover rate and rapid muscle growth, it is also important to have a positive caloric balance; in other words, to consume more calories than you expend. There exists substantial evidence indicating that strength athletes can increase muscle mass and strength by simply increasing their caloric consumption. Moreover, there is substantial evidence indicating that a negative caloric balance (consuming fewer calories than are expended) will adversely affect nitrogen retention.

As early as 1907, it was reported that athletes gained strength and maintained mass on relatively low-protein diets as long as sufficient calories were consumed. In addition, a positive caloric balance as compared to an equal caloric balance has been shown to produce the greater gains in muscle mass in subjects undergoing resistance training. Therefore, to maximize your gains in muscle mass, construct your diet so that you consume more calories than you expend.

NTS RECOMMENDATIONS FOR THE GROWTH PHASE

A fundamental principle of the Nutrient Timing System is metabolic sensitivity. By now it should be apparent that the metabolic action of a particular nutrient is highly dependent on when it is consumed. The concept of metabolic sensitivity is illustrated clearly in the nutrient recommendations for this phase.

A carbohydrate/protein supplement is necessary to maintain the anabolic state and heightened level of insulin sensitivity in the four-hour period after your workout. However, once the insulin pump has been primed, less carbohydrate is needed to maintain elevated insulin levels. Whereas a carbohydrate/protein mixture containing more carbohydrate relative to protein (such as 3 to 4 grams of carbohydrate to 1 gram of protein) is ideal to turn on the anabolic machinery, supplementation during the Rapid Segment can rely on a much lower carbohydrate to protein ratio. In fact, 1 gram of carbohydrate to 5–8 grams of protein is appropriate.

Carbohydrate is still needed in amounts sufficient to keep the insulin pump operating at its optimum level. On the other hand, if too much carbohydrate is consumed, it can be converted into fat. Keeping the insulin level elevated for a sustained four-hour period prevents development of insulin resistance, which, as we have seen, will slow or turn off those metabolic processes that are critical for building muscle mass and strength.

It is also recommended that during the Rapid Segment you consume leucine and glutamine because of their anabolic action on protein synthesis and immune system parameters. Table 5.2 describes the ideal nutrient composition for a supplement to be used during the Rapid Segment. This nutrient composition will help maintain the high anabolic activity initiated during the Anabolic Phase.

During the Sustained Segment of the Growth Phase, insulin levels decline, but it is possible to sustain protein synthesis, although at a slower rate than during the Rapid Segment. This can be accomplished with a proper diet and a carbohydrate/protein snack between meals.

Because your diet represents the bulk of your caloric intake, it has the most influence on protein synthesis and muscle growth during the Sustained Segment.

TABLE 5.2. Ideal Nutrient Composition of Supplement for the Growth Phase

GROWTH PHASE	NTS Objective	Nutrient	Amount
Rapid Segment The first 4 hours after a workout	• Maintain increased insulin sensitivity	Whey protein	14 g
	• Maintain the anabolic state	Casein	2 g
Sustained Segment The next 16–18 hours after a workout	• Maintain positive nitrogen balance and stimulate protein synthesis	Leucine	3 g
		Glutamine	1 g
	• Promote protein turnover and muscle development	High-glycemic carbohydrates	2–4 g

The supplement recommended for the Rapid Segment of the Growth Phase is a high-protein snack that can be used between meals and at bedtime during the Sustained Segment. Such a protein snack or supplement enables you to stimulate protein synthesis by raising the amino acid levels in your blood between meals. As we have shown, elevated amino acid levels stimulate protein synthesis and also slow protein degradation, thereby increasing your net protein balance.

Most important, the high-protein snack does not stimulate insulin. Whereas insulin is essential at specific times, continued elevation of insulin along with high-carbohydrate consumption is not desirable. This insulin elevation can lead to increased fat deposition, elevated blood cholesterol levels, and metabolic disorders.

Protein Type

The objective during both segments of the Growth Phase is to maintain protein synthesis over an extended period of time. Selection of the right type of protein can help you achieve this goal. When comparing the proteins whey and casein, investigators found that protein synthesis increased 68 percent with a whey supplement and 32 percent with a casein supplement. However, the anabolic response of the casein was longer lasting. Because whey is fast acting and the effects of casein are more sustained, we recommend taking a supplement snack composed of both whey and casein during the Growth Phase.

Caloric Balance

Your diet should be in positive caloric balance for muscle repair and growth to be optimized. How large a positive caloric balance will depend on your goals. If you are just trying to gain strength without trying to add much weight, your caloric intake should only exceed your caloric expenditure by 50–100 calories per day. If you are trying to increase mass, you may want your caloric intake to exceed your caloric expenditure by several hundred calories per day. However, if you are a bodybuilder in preparation for competition, you will want to have a negative caloric balance for several weeks leading up to the competition in order to reduce body fat. During this time, you should reduce your carbohydrate intake and increase your protein intake. Table 5.3 summarizes general caloric and nutrient recommendations depending on your specific training goals. However, these are general guidelines. If you find you are not getting the results you want, don't assume that your genes are working against you. If your goal is to gain muscle mass and you are consuming an extra 100–200 calories per day and are not seeing positive results, simply increase your daily caloric intake by another 100–200 calories.

TABLE 5.3. Daily Caloric Consumption and Macronutrient Content Based on Exercise Goals

Goal	Daily Caloric Balance	Protein	Carbohydrate	Fat
Gain strength	plus 50–100 calories	21–24%	43–46%	33%
Gain lean mass	plus 100–200 calories	21–24%	43–46%	33%
Decrease fat mass	minus 100–200 calories	26%	41%	33%

Making Nutrient Timing Work for You

Sports nutrition is skewed toward two ends of the information spectrum. At one end are the nutritionists and "nutritional experts" who advocate a 1960s approach to sports nutrition. Their advice consists mainly of paying attention to the food pyramid, eating lots of leafy vegetables, and trying to control fat intake. According to this approach, you should get all the nutrients you need by following a healthy diet. At the other end of the spectrum are the sports nutrition companies who are often the purveyors of hype. These are the manufacturers who claim their products will "double your lean body mass in a week" while extolling the virtues of their magic herbs and supplements. For them, product claims tend to come out of a thesaurus rather than from a research laboratory. They are the advocates of "more is better." If an ingredient has a benefit, then more of it will give you a greater benefit. Ironically, both of these groups take a similar view of current nutrition research.

For many nutrition traditionalists, good scientific research ended around 1980. They generally fail to incorporate in their programs some of the landmark studies showing how nutrition could have improved the sports performances of the last two decades.

For the purveyors of hype, good scientific research is remote. Their product claims are usually not substantiated by studies, and when they are, the studies may not be relevant to the modern-day athlete's realities.

This information abyss presents a true challenge for the serious strength athlete as he or she tries to navigate through hype and outdated thinking. And of course, most serious athletes are not usually trained in exercise physiology.

We have cited many studies showing the significant and dramatic gains in muscle strength and development that you can achieve by applying a few basic nutrition principles. The science supporting Nutrient Timing is growing; our extensive bibliography at the end of this book is evidence of this growth.

As scientists who are committed to finding safe ways to help improve athletic performance, we find that the most exciting aspect of Nutrient Timing is its power as a tool to help strength athletes achieve their full athletic potential. Figure 6.1 clearly shows the negative impact of nutrient procrastination on most of the muscle cells' key anabolic activities. It also illustrates the positive impact of timely nutrient consumption. Among its other effects, a carbohydrate/protein supplement taken immediately after exercise (versus waiting up to three hours) can result in a

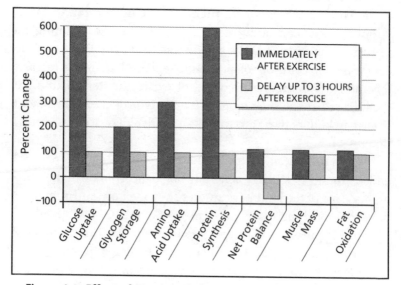

Figure 6.1. Effect of Nutrient Delay on Key Anabolic Activities

600 percent improvement in protein synthesis and a 100 percent improvement in muscle glycogen replenishment. Following the principles of Nutrient Timing will provide you with the kind of results that will be as powerful as, if not more powerful than, any other sports nutrition program or product.

However, no matter how strong the science, it must be practical. In other words, Nutrient Timing has to work in the training regimens of strength athletes at all levels and every day. Many pages of this book have been devoted to discussing the science underlying the three phases of Nutrient Timing. In this chapter, we fulfill the promise we made in the Introduction. Nutrient Timing is a practical and easy program to implement.

The nutrition foundation for Nutrient Timing is a healthy diet. We offer a number of dietary suggestions and, most important, we have created a template so you can design your own diet based on your own tastes, habits, and lifestyle. To this nutrition foundation, we have added nutrient intervention at three critical times in the muscles' growth cycle: the Energy Phase, the Anabolic Phase, and the Rapid Segment of the Growth Phase. This additional supplementation is usually in the form of a beverage; however, with the exception of the Energy Phase in which hydration is so important, you can create your Anabolic and Growth Phase supplements with the right combination of solid foods. As discussed, there are a number of advantages in taking your nutritional supplementation as a beverage during the four-hour time span that begins just prior to your workout and ends two to three hours after your workout.

The macronutrient requirements for strength athletes looking to get the most out of Nutrient Timing are as follows:

- 19 to 26 percent protein

- 41 to 48 percent carbohydrate

- 33 percent fat

For strength athletes, protein consumption of 0.9–1.2 grams of protein per pound of body weight is ideal. This diet will give you the extra protein you need, which, as we have seen, can help enhance muscle development as well as the necessary energy from carbohydrate and fat to maintain a healthy immune system and minimize the development of overtraining syndrome.

Table 6.1 shows the nutrient composition at different levels of protein intake for a male weighing 200 pounds and a female weighing 130 pounds.

TABLE 6.1. Daily Nutrient Compositions at Four Levels of Protein Intake

MALE • Weight: 200 pounds • Target Daily Caloric Intake: 3,800

Protein Level (g/lb)	Protein Composition			Carbohydrate Composition			Fat Composition		
	Calories	Grams	Percent	Calories	Grams	Percent	Calories	Grams	Percent
0.09	728	182	19	1,818	455	48	1,254	139	33
1.02	816	204	21	1,730	433	46	1,254	139	33
1.14	912	228	24	1,634	409	43	1,254	139	33
1.25	1,000	250	26	1,564	387	41	1,254	139	33

FEMALE • Weight: 130 pounds • Target Daily Caloric Intake: 2,340

Protein Level (g/lb)	Protein Composition			Carbohydrate Composition			Fat Composition		
	Calories	Grams	Percent	Calories	Grams	Percent	Calories	Grams	Percent
0.09	473	118	20	1,095	274	47	772	86	33
1.02	532	133	23	1,036	259	44	772	86	33
1.14	591	148	25	977	244	42	772	86	33
1.25	650	163	28	918	229	39	772	86	33

3 + 1—The Secret for Implementing Nutrient Timing

Three plus one is all it takes to get the full benefits of Nutrient

Timing—that is, nutrient intervention three times around your workout plus one healthy diet. As shown in Table 6.2, you also have the option of taking another growth phase supplement as a post-dinner snack to achieve greater muscle growth.

Table 6.2 outlines a sample food plan for a 200-pound strength athlete who works out once per day. The goal protein level is 1.1 gram per pound for a daily total of 228 grams. As you can see, it is not a complex program. However, it does require paying special attention to nutrition during the periods when your muscles are most susceptible to damage and when they are most susceptible to growth. This may mean a slight change in your eating habits.

TABLE 6.2. Daily Caloric Composition for a 200-Pound Male Athlete Who Works Out Once Daily

The goal protein amount is 228 grams; the goal caloric intake is 3,800 calories.

	Protein	Carbohydrate	Fat	Calories
Breakfast	28 g	80 g	28 g	684
Workout (Energy Supplement)	6 g	24 g	1 g	129
Postworkout (Anabolic Supplement)	15 g	45 g	1 g	249
2 Hours Postworkout (Growth Supplement)	20 g	4 g	1 g	105
Lunch	46 g	82 g	18 g	674
Snack	14 g	92 g	33 g	721
Dinner	56 g	80 g	49 g	985
Post-dinner (Growth Supplement)	20 g	4 g	1 g	105
TOTAL	226 g	411 g	138 g	3,790

In our examples, we have scheduled your workout in the morning. We recognize that with busy schedules athletes do not have a set time each day for their workout. To implement the Nutrient Timing System, you do not have to perform a morning workout. However, whenever your workout occurs, it is important that you consume the proper nutrients during the three critical phases. If need be, adjust your meals accordingly.

Table 6.3 summarizes the ideal nutrient composition for each phase of the Nutrient Timing System. As mentioned previously, the ideal form for the NTS supplement in the Energy Phase is a beverage, which will help replace fluids lost during your workout. Although there are many advantages to consuming a beverage for the Anabolic and Growth Phase, solid food can work just as well as long as the nutrient composition is optimal.

TABLE 6.3. NTS Recommended Supplements Nutrient Profile

NTS PHASE	NTS Objective	Nutrient	Amount
ENERGY PHASE 10 minutes prior to and during a workout	• Increase nutrient delivery to muscles and spare muscle glycogen and protein • Limit immune system suppression • Minimize muscle damage • Set the nutritional stage for a faster recovery following your workout	High-glycemic carbohydrates (glucose, sucrose, and maltodextrin)	20–26 g
		Whey protein	5–6 g
		Leucine	1 g
		Vitamin C	30–120 mg
		Vitamin E	20–60 IU
		Sodium	100–250 IU
		Potassium	60–120 mg
		Magnesium	60–120 mg
ANABOLIC PHASE Within 45 minutes after a workout	• Shift metabolic machinery from a catabolic state to an anabolic state • Speed the elimination of metabolic wastes by increasing muscle blood flow • Replenish muscle glycogen stores • Initiate tissue repair and set the stage for muscle growth • Reduce muscle damage and bolster the immune system	Whey protein	13–15 g
		High-glycemic carbohydrates (glucose, sucrose, and maltodextrin)	40–50 g
		Leucine	1–2 g
		Glutamine	1–2 g
		Vitamin C	60–120 mg
		Vitamin E	80–400 IU
GROWTH PHASE	**Rapid Segment** The first 4 hours after a workout • Maintain increased insulin sensitivity • Maintain the anabolic state	Whey protein	14 g
		Casein	2 g
		Leucine	3 g
	Sustained Segment The next 16–18 hours after a workout • Maintain positive nitrogen balance and stimulate protein synthesis • Promote protein turnover and muscle development	Glutamine	1 g
		High-glycemic carbohydrates	2–4 g

Conclusion

When the first studies that lay the groundwork for the Nutrient Timing System were published, they were met with skepticism by many exercise physiologists and nutritionists. There have now been many studies conducted worldwide that support the science underlying the Nutrient Timing System. Additional studies are essential if we are to fully understand the mechanisms by which nutrition can influence muscle cell growth. It is clear that strength athletes, and, in fact, all athletes, trainers, strength and conditioning coaches, and nutritionists will benefit by adopting the Nutrient Timing System. Finally, the Nutrient Timing System gives us a tool that will enable athletes to safely achieve gains in strength, power, and performance with the most basic of all tools—the food they eat.

Selected References

Andersen, J.L., Schjerling, P., Andersen, L.L., and Dela, F., "Resistance training and insulin action in humans: effects of de-training," *Journal of Physiology*, 551: 1049–1058, 2003.

Anthony, J.C., Anthony, T.G., and Layman, D.K., "Leucine supplementation enhances skeletal muscle recovery in rats following exercise," *Journal of Nutrition*, 129: 1102–1106, 1999.

Baron, A.D., Steinberg, H., Brechtel, G., et al., "Skeletal muscle blood flow independently modulates insulin-mediated glucose uptake," *American Journal of Physiology*, 266: E248–E253, 1994.

Biolo, G., Tipton, K.D., Klein, S., et al., "An abundant supply of amino acids enhances the metabolic effect of exercise on muscle protein," *American Journal of Physiology*, 273: E122–E119, 1997.

Bishop, N.C., Blannin, A.K., Rand, L., et al., "Effects of carbohydrate and fluid intake on the blood leukocyte responses to prolonged cycling," *International Journal of Sport Medicine*, 17: 26–27, 1999.

Bishop, N.C., Blannin, A.K., Rand, L., et al., "The effects of carbohydrate supplementation on neutrophil degranulation responses to prolonged cycling," *International Journal of Sport Medicine*, 21(Suppl 1): S73, 2000.

Bishop, N.C., Blannin, A.K., Walsh, N.P., et al., "Carbohydrate beverage ingestion and neutrophil degranulation responses following cycling to fatigue at 75% VO2 max," *International Journal of Sport Medicine*, 22: 226–231, 2001.

Blom, P.C.S., Høstmark, A.T., Vaage, O., et al., "Effect of different post-exercise sugar diets on the rate of muscle glycogen synthesis," *Medicine and Science in Sports and Exercise*, 19: 491–496, 1987.

Blomstrand, E., and Saltin B., "BCAA intake affects protein metabolism in muscle after but not during exercise in human," *American Journal of Physiology*, 28: E365–E374, 2001.

Boirie, Y., Dangin, M., Gachon, P., et al., "Slow and fast dietary proteins differently modulate postprandial protein accretion," *Proceedings of the National Academy of Sciences, USA*, 94: 14930–12935, 1997.

Cardillo, C., Kilcoyne, C.M., Nambi, S.S., et al., "Vasodilator response to systemic but not to local hyperinsulemia in the human forearm," *Hypertension*, 34: E12–E13, 1999.

Chandler, R.M., Byrne, H.K., Patterson, J.G., and Ivy, J.L., "Dietary supplements affect the anabolic hormones after high resistance exercise," *Journal of Applied Physiology*, 76: 839–845, 1994.

Chittenden, R.H., The Nutrition of Man. Heinemann, London, 1907.

Cumming, D.C., Wall, S.R., Galbraith, M.A., and Belcastro, A.N., "Reproductive hormonal responses to resistance exercise," *Medicine and Science in Sports and Exercise*, 19: 234–238, 1987.

Esmarck, B., Andersen, J.L., Olsen, S., et al., "Timing of post exercise protein intake is important for muscle hypertrophy with resistance training in elderly humans," *Journal of Physiology*, 535: 301–311, 2001.

Evans, W.J., "Protein nutrition and resistance exercise," *Canadian Journal of Applied Physiology*, 26 (Suppl): S141–S152, 2001.

Fern, E.B., Bielinski, R.N., and Schutz, Y., "Effects of exaggerated amino acid and protein supply in man," *Experientia*, 47: 168–172, 1991.

Fielding, R.A., and Parkington, J., "What are the dietary protein requirements of physically active individuals? New evidence on the effects of exercise on protein utilization during postexercise recovery," *Nutrition and Clinical Care*, 5: 191–196, 2002.

Flakoll, P.J., Judy, T., Flinn, K., Carr, C., and Flinn, S. "Post-exercise protein supplementation improves health and muscle soreness during basic military training in marine recruits," *Journal of Applied Physiology*, 96: 951–956, 2004.

Forslund, A.H., El-Khoury, A.E., Olsson, R.M., et al., "Effect of protein intake and physical activity on 24-h pattern and rate of macronutrient utilization," *American Journal or Physiology*, 276: E964–E976, 1999.

Forslund, A.H., Habraeus, L., Olsson, R.M., et al., "The 24-h whole body leucine and urea kinetics at normal and high protein intake with exercise in healthy adults," *American Journal of Physiology*, 275: E310–E320, 1998.

Forslund, A.H., Habraeus, L., Van Beurden, H., et al., "Inverse relationship between protein intake and plasma free amino acids in healthy men at physical exercise," *American Journal of Physiology*, 278: E857–E867, 2000.

Gater, D.R., Gater, D.A., Uribe, J.M., et al., "Impact of nutritional supplements and resistance training on body composition, strength and insulin-like growth factor-1," *Journal of Applied Sports Science Research*, 6: 66–76, 1992.

Gleeson, M., Lancaster, G.I., and Bishop, N.C., "Nutritional strategies to minimize exercise-induced immunosuppression in athletes," *Canadian Journal of Applied Physiology*, 26 (Suppl): S23–S35, 2001.

Haff, G.G., Koch, A.J, Potteiger, J.A., et al., "Carbohydrate supplementation attenuates muscle glycogen loss during acute bouts of resistance exercise," *International Journal of Sport Nutrition and Exercise Metabolism*, 10: 326–339, 2000.

Haff, G.G., Lehmkuhl, M.J., McCoy, L.B., et al., "Carbohydrate supplementation and resistance training," *Journal of Strength and Conditioning Research*, 17: 187–196, 2003.

Ivy, J.L., "Dietary strategies to promote glycogen synthesis after exercise," *Canadian Journal of Applied Physiology*, 26 (Suppl): S236–S245, 2001.

Ivy, J.L., Goforth, H.W., Jr., Damon, B.M., et al., "Early post exercise muscle glycogen recovery is enhanced with a carbohydrate-protein supplement," *Journal of Applied Physiology*, 93: 1337–1344, 2002.

Ivy, J.L., Katz, A.L., Cutler, C.L., et al., "Muscle glycogen synthesis after exercise: effect of time on carbohydrate ingestion," *Journal of Applied Physiology*, 64: 1480–1485, 1988.

Ivy, J.L., Lee, M.C., Brozinick, J.T., et al., "Muscle glycogen storage after different amounts of carbohydrate ingestion," *Journal of Applied Physiology*, 65: 2018–2023, 1988.

Ivy, J.L., Res, P.T., Sprague, R.C., et al., "Effect of carbohydrate-protein supplement on endurance performance during exercise of varying intensity," *International Journal of Sport Nutrition and Exercise Metabolism*, 13: 388–401, 2003.

Kraemer, W.J., "Endocrine responses to resistance exercise," *Medicine and Science in Sports and Exercise*, 20: S152–S157, 1988.

Kraemer, W.J., Marchitelli, L., Gordon, S.E., et al., "Hormonal and growth factor responses to heavy resistance exercise protocols," *Journal of Applied Physiology*, 69: 1442–50, 1990.

Laakso, M., Edelman, S.V., Brechtel, G., and Baron, A.D., "Decreased effect of insulin to stimulate skeletal muscle blood flow in obese man: a novel mechanism for insulin resistance," *Journal of Clinical Investigation*, 85: 1844–1852, 1990.

Lemon, P.W., Dolny, D.G., Yarasheski, K.E., "Moderate physical activity can increase dietary protein needs," *Canadian Journal of Applied Physiology*, 22: 494–503, 1997.

Levenhagen, D.K., Carr, C., Carlson, M.G., et al., "Post exercise protein intake enhances whole-body and leg protein accretion in humans," *Medicine and Science in Sports and Exercise*, 34: 828–837, 2002.

Levenhagen, D.K., Gresham, J.D., Carlson, M.G., et al., "Post exercise nutrient intake timing in humans is critical to recovery of leg glucose and protein homeostasis," *American Journal Physiology*, 280: E982–E993, 2001.

Miller, S.L., Tipton, K.D., Chinkes, D.L., et al., "Independent and combined effects of amino acids and glucose after resistance exercise," *Medicine and Science in Sports and Exercise*, 35: 449–455, 2003.

Miller, W.J., Sherman, W.M., and Ivy, J.L., "Effect of strength training on glucose tolerance and post glucose insulin response," *Medicine and Science in Sports and Exercise*, 16: 539–543, 1984.

National Academy of Sciences National Research Council, Recommended Dietary Allowances, (9th edition), Washington, D.C.: National Academy Press, 1989.

Nieman, D.C., Johansen, L.M., Lee, J.W., et al., "Infectious episodes in runners before and after the Los Angeles Marathon," *Journal of Sports Medicine and Physical Fitness*, 30: 316–328, 1990.

Okamura, K., Doi, T., Hamada, K., et al., "Effect of amino acid and glucose administration during postexercise recovery on protein kinetics in dogs," *American Journal of Physiology*," 272: E1023–E1030, 1997.

Rasmussen, B.B., Tipton, K.D., Miller, S.L., et al., "An oral essential amino acid-carbohydrate supplement enhances muscle protein anabolism after resistance exercise," *Journal of Applied Physiology*, 88: 386–392, 2000.

Ready, S.L., Seifert, J., Burke, E., "Effect of two sports drinks on muscle tissue stress and performance," *Medicine and Science in Sports and Exercise*, 31(5): S119, 1999.

Rokitzki, L., Logeman, E., Sagredos, A.N., et al., "Lipid peroxidation and antioxidant vitamins under extreme endurance stress," *Acta Physiologica Scandinavacia*, 151: 149–158, 1994.

Rokitzki, L., Logemann, E., Huber, G., et al., "Alpha-Tocopherol supplementation in racing cyclists during extreme endurance training," *International Journal of Sport Nutrition*, 4: 253–264, 1994.

Roy, B.D., Fowles, J.R., Hill, R., et al., "Macronutrient intake and whole body protein metabolism following resistance exercise," *Medicine and Science in Sports and Exercise*, 32: 1412–1418, 2000.

Spiller, G.A., Jensen, C.D., Pattison, T.S., et al., "Effect of protein dose on serum glucose and insulin response to sugars," *American Journal of Clinical Nutrition*, 46: 474–481, 1987.

Suzuki, M., Doi, T., Lee, S.J., et al., "Effect of meal timing after resistance exercise on hind limb muscle mass and fat accumulation in trained rats," *Journal of Nutritional Science and Vitaminology*, 45: 401–409, 1999.

Tarnopolsky, M.A., "Protein and physical performance," *Current Opinions on Clinical Nutrition and Metabolic Care*, 2: 533–537, 1999.

Tarnopolsky, M.A., Atkinson, S.A., MacDougall, J.D., et al., "Whole body leucine metabolism during and after resistance exercise in fed humans," *Medicine and Science in Sports and Exercise*, 23: 326–333, 1991.

Tarnopolsky, M.A., Bosman, M., MacDonald, J.R., et al., "Post exercise protein-carbohydrate and carbohydrate supplements increase muscle glycogen in men and women," *Journal of Applied Physiology*, 83: 1877–1883, 1997.

Tarnopolsky, M.A., MacDougall, J.D., Atkinson, S.A., "Influence of protein intake and training status on nitrogen balance and lean body mass," *Journal of Applied Physiology*, 64: 187–193, 1988.

van der Schoor, P., van Hall, G., Saris, W.H.M., et al., "Ingestion of protein hydrolysate prevents the post-exercise reduction in plasma glutamate," *International Journal of Sports Medicine*, 18: S115, 1997.

Van Loon, L.J., Saris, W.H.M., Kruijshoop, M., et al., "Maximizing post exercise muscle glycogen synthesis: carbohydrate supplementation and the application of amino acid or protein hydrolysate mixtures," *American Journal of Clinical Nutrition*, 72: 106–111, 2000.

Van Loon, L.J.C., Saris, W.H.M., Verhagen, H., et al., "Plasma insulin responses following the ingestion of different amino acid and/or protein mixtures with carbohydrate," *American Journal of Clinical Nutrition*, 72: 96–105, 2000.

Williams, M., Ivy, J., Raven, P., "Effects of recovery drinks after prolonged glycogen-depletion exercise," *Medicine and Science in Sports and Exercise*, 31(5):S124, 1999.

Williams, M.B., Raven, P.B., Donovan L.F., et al., "Effects of recovery beverage on glycogen restoration and endurance exercise performance," *Journal of Strength and Conditioning Research*, 17: 12–19, 2003.

Yaspelkis, B.B., Patterson, J.G., Anderla, P.A., et al., "Carbohydrate supplementation spares muscle glycogen during variable-intensity exercise," *Journal of Applied Physiology*, 75: 1477–1485, 1993.

Zawadzki, K.M., Yaspelkis, B.B., III, and Ivy, J.L., "Carbohydrate-protein complex increases the rate of muscle glycogen storage after exercise," *Journal of Applied Physiology*, 72: 1854–1859, 1992.

Index

About the Authors

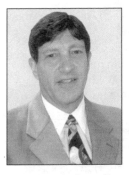

John Ivy is Chair and Margie Gurley Seay Centennial Professor in the Department of Kinesiology & Health Education at the University of Texas at Austin. He received his Ph.D. in Exercise Physiology from the University of Maryland and his post-doctoral training in physiology and biochemistry from Washington University School of Medicine. He has published over 150 research papers on the effects of nutrition on physical performance and exercise recovery. He is a Fellow and former Ambassador for the American College of Sports Medicine and Fellow in the American Academy of Kinesiology.

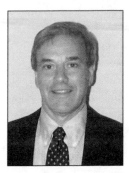

Robert Portman earned his Ph.D. in biochemistry from Virginia Tech. He has numerous scientific publications and has written and lectured extensively on the role of nutrition in improving exercise performance. Dr. Portman is head of research at PacificHealth Laboratories, a nutrition technology company that has pioneered in the development of innovative nutritional products to help athletes reach their potential.

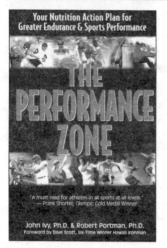